# THE COVID-19
# INTELLIGENCE
# FAILURE

# THE COVID-19 INTELLIGENCE FAILURE

WHY WARNING WAS NOT ENOUGH

ERIK J. DAHL

GEORGETOWN UNIVERSITY PRESS / WASHINGTON, DC

The publisher is not responsible for third-party websites or their content. URL links were active at time of publication.

Library of Congress Cataloging-in-Publication Data

Names: Dahl, Erik J., author.
Title: The covid-19 intelligence failure: why warning was not enough / Erik J. Dahl.
Description: Washington, DC: Georgetown University Press, 2023. | Includes
    bibliographical references and index.
Identifiers: LCCN 2022005425 (print) | LCCN 2022005426 (ebook) |
    ISBN 9781647123055 (hardcover) | ISBN 9781647123062 (paperback) |
    ISBN 9781647123079 (ebook)
Subjects: LCSH: COVID-19 (Disease) | Public health surveillance. | Pandemics. |
    Intelligence service—United States. | Public health—United States.
Classification: LCC RA644.C67 D335 2023 (print) | LCC RA644.C67 (ebook) |
    DDC 614.5/92414—dc23/eng/20220218
LC record available at https://lccn.loc.gov/2022005425
LC ebook record available at https://lccn.loc.gov/2022005426

♾ This paper meets the requirements of ANSI/NISO Z39.48-1992 (Permanence of Paper).

24  23      9 8 7 6 5 4 3 2 First printing

Printed in the United States of America

Cover design by Jeremy John Parker
Interior design by BookComp, Inc.
Production Assistant, Jenna Galberg

# CONTENTS

# CONTENTS

# ACKNOWLEDGMENTS

Early in 2020, when the world began to lock down because of the coronavirus outbreak, I was struck by a puzzle: How was it possible that we were taken by surprise by the virus, when for years experts had been warning about the threat of just this kind of global pandemic? I realized that many of the questions being discussed around the world, such as how to assess the threat and how best to gather data on the spread of the disease, were the same questions asked routinely of intelligence professionals.

I wanted to understand how the COVID-19 pandemic could have happened. At first it seemed like an impossible task to write a book that would examine the crisis from the perspective of both traditional national security intelligence and medical and public health intelligence and warning. Thanks to the support, advice, and encouragement of many colleagues, friends, and experts in a number of fields, this book is the result.

My colleagues in the National Security Affairs Department at the Naval Postgraduate School have been extremely helpful and supportive, and I would especially like to thank Alex Matovski, Tom Bruneau, and Emily Meierding for providing very helpful comments on the book proposal; Jim Wirtz, for facilitating my presentation of that proposal to the National Security Affairs Department faculty research colloquium and for providing extensive comments; Zach Shore, for reading and giving excellent advice on several chapters; and Maria Rasmussen, for being extremely supportive throughout.

I presented early versions of several chapters to the Canadian Association for Security and Intelligence Studies, to a workshop hosted by Defence Research and Development Canada, at several events sponsored by the Center for Homeland Defense and Security, and at the 2021 International Studies Association annual conference. I was able to develop my thinking about the pandemic and intelligence in articles that appeared in *The Duck of Minerva*, *The Conversation*, and *Homeland Security Affairs*.

For providing advice and encouragement I would like to thank Javed Ali, Michael Brody, Matt Dolan, Steve Park, and Brian Powers. I would especially like to thank Victoria Clement, Joe Faragone, John Gentry, Jennifer

Hughes-Large, Jay Mercer, William Pilkington, Patrick Walsh, Wesley Wark, James Wilson, and David Young, all of whom provided extensive comments and took time for lengthy discussions by email, on Zoom, or through other virtual platforms. Don Jacobs, my editor at Georgetown University Press, has been, once again, greatly supportive. The press's anonymous reviewers provided very helpful comments on the proposal and on the final manuscript. The views expressed in this book are my own and do not represent the views of the US government or the Naval Postgraduate School.

This book is dedicated to my wonderful wife, Christa.

# INTRODUCTION

## Intelligence, Warning, and Disaster

William Farr, a British physician who was an important figure early in the field of epidemiology, wrote about a cholera epidemic that struck the United Kingdom in 1848–49:

> If a foreign army had landed on the coast of England, seized all the seaports . . . ravaged the population through the summer and . . . in the year it held possession of the country slain fifty-three thousand two hundred and ninety-three men, women and children, . . . the task of registering the dead would be inexpressibly painful; and the pain is not greatly diminished by the circumstance that in the calamity to be described the minister of destruction was a pestilence.[1]

In late 2019 and 2020 an "army" landed in the United States and in almost every other inhabited part of the globe. As happened in William Farr's Britain, the invader was not an army of soldiers. It was a virus—one that killed more in the United States than both world wars and the Vietnam War combined.[2]

This book examines the roles that intelligence, surveillance, and warning play in the fight against COVID-19 and other global health threats.[3] It attempts to answer questions such as: Are pandemic threats purely a health concern, or are they a national security problem? What is the role of traditional national security intelligence agencies in warning and tracking the development of an outbreak? How does the work of intelligence differ from the work performed by international and domestic medical intelligence and surveillance systems? Was the coronavirus pandemic an intelligence failure and, if it was, how can our intelligence and warning systems be improved so that we can anticipate, detect, and respond more effectively to the next pandemic surely to arise?

My focus is primarily on the US intelligence community (IC) and the experiences during the COVID-19 pandemic in the United States. But because this pandemic has affected nearly the entire globe and involves a myriad of national and international medical and public health organizations, it also provides the opportunity to conduct an in-depth review of the many medical surveillance

1

systems that have been established to detect and warn about infectious disease outbreaks and allows a comparison of the US experience with that of other nations.

Why the comparison between traditional national security intelligence and medical intelligence? In part this approach is appropriate because these two fields use much of the same language and many of the same concepts when gathering information. For example, in both national security and public health, analysts are faced with the problem of having many more "signals" of possible threats than they can focus on. Some experts have argued that the process of disease surveillance, which is critical for tracking and limiting the spread of an epidemic, closely resembles the intelligence cycle that has long been taught to budding intelligence analysts. These two fields also give rise to similar concerns about the potential harm that intelligence programs can do when they encroach on civil liberties and personal freedoms; for example, critics have warned that the pandemic may lead to overbearing surveillance in the future, such as through the use of contact-tracing phone apps.[4]

Most important, we need to discuss both national security and medical intelligence together because the two fields naturally overlap: a traditional national security analyst must be familiar with the tools and techniques of medical intelligence and surveillance in order to be able to analyze disease threats, and senior-level public health professionals will be able to advise decision-makers only if they understand and can assess the other streams of information that will be coming in during a pandemic. As we have seen with the coronavirus and with previous disease outbreaks, effective intelligence and warning must involve all hands and all professions.

It may seem presumptuous for an intelligence scholar and former practitioner to attempt to offer advice to professionals in the fields of medicine and public health. After all, the profession of national security intelligence has not yet learned how to avoid failure and surprise. But intelligence experts have long noted the similarities between their work and that of medicine. Walter Laqueur, for example, wrote that "the student of intelligence will profit more from contemplating the principles of medical diagnosis than immersing himself in any other field."[5] Medical and public health experts frequently compare the work they do to the work performed by intelligence analysts (discussed in chapter 3). Yet, despite these similarities, the fields of intelligence, medicine, and public health too often remain disconnected from each other. This book is one of the first to provide an in-depth analysis of the roles that both traditional intelligence services and medical intelligence and surveillance systems played in the COVID-19 pandemic.

In this book "intelligence" is defined broadly and not just consisting of the secret information that is normally associated with the term. Intelligence is a process—and a function of government and society—that involves gathering information, assessing its significance, and presenting those assessments to decision-makers. David Omand, the former security and intelligence coordinator for the British government and former director of Government Communications Headquarters (GCHQ), the British version of the US National Security Agency (NSA), offers a useful definition of the role of intelligence: "The purpose of having intelligence is to enable better, more timely, decisions by reducing the ignorance of the decision takers."[6] Today, more than ever before, we find that the information and warning needed by decision-makers at all levels of government can come from many different sources, and it is no longer appropriate—if it ever was—to think of intelligence as only coming from secretive, three-letter agencies. As a number of experts have noted, the current crisis has demonstrated the critical need for what is termed "open-source" or unclassified intelligence, whether that intelligence is gathered by a traditional intelligence agency, a public-health-surveillance system, or a new source that may still need to be developed.[7]

## THE PURPOSE OF THIS BOOK

This assessment brings together the fields of intelligence, medicine, and public health to help these different communities understand each other. This is no easy task, because these communities see the world very differently and may not be inclined to coordinate or even talk with each other. As described by Kenneth W. Bernard, a former assistant US surgeon general and advisor to the National Security Council (NSC), public health and national security are like two tribes that find it difficult to trust each other. National security specialists may not see health as their core business, while "public health experts often are reluctant to trust those in the security community they see as coming from the 'dark side.'"[8] Tara O'Toole, a medical doctor and public health expert who has worked closely with the intelligence community, notes that US intelligence agencies have not typically considered health issues to be a part of national security.[9] But it is vital that these communities work together.

This analysis has a broader goal as well: to help all of us use intelligence more effectively to prevent threats to society, including but not limited to health threats such as pandemics. Experts have noted a lack of knowledge about health subjects on the part of US national security decision-makers, and called for new and better ways to collect, analyze, and disseminate information and intelligence on global disease threats.[10] I hope this book provides some of the knowledge needed by policymakers and advances the national and global discussion about how to improve the disease and health intelligence and warning system. While the next global crisis might come in the form of another pandemic, it also could develop from a very different source, such as global climate change. The book's conclusion examines how the intelligence lessons from the COVID-19 pandemic may also be useful in helping anticipate and avoid other kinds of threats.

## THE CONTRIBUTION OF THIS BOOK

This book makes four specific contributions. First, it explains the roles and functions of the traditional intelligence community in the areas of health and disease and of the medical and public health communities in terms of intelligence and surveillance. Second, it tells the story of how these communities functioned during the COVID-19 pandemic. This book will not be the last word on this history, especially if, as I hope, there will be a future national coronavirus commission in the United States and similar international investigative bodies. Enough information is now available to enable us to tell a relatively complete story and help us understand and remember the lessons from the current crisis.

Third, this analysis goes beyond the facts and history of the current crisis to make an argument about how well intelligence, surveillance, and warning have performed. This involves judgments about questions that can have no absolute right or wrong answer, such as whether intelligence and warning could have been better than it was. Such assessments must be made if we hope to learn lessons from the pandemic.

Fourth, and finally, I make recommendations for how we might do better next time. Many experts have noted that this pandemic could have been much worse—the next one, as Michael T. Osterholm and Mark Olshaker write, "could really be 'the Big One,' and it could make even the current pandemic seem minor by comparison."[11] If we hope to prevent such a future disaster we must begin to improve our intelligence and warning capabilities now.

## THE CASE FOR CHANGE

Debates about intelligence and the coronavirus have focused mostly on whether the US intelligence community did a good job of reporting on the outbreak, or on how the Donald Trump administration failed to heed the early warnings. These debates are important, but they miss the larger point about intelligence and the coronavirus pandemic. Earlier detection of the outbreak and better understanding of its significance could have accelerated the international response and reduced the human toll and economic costs associated with the virus, but our existing systems of intelligence and surveillance were insufficient. The pandemic was a global intelligence failure in which the complex worldwide system of collection, analysis, and warning that had been developed to address just this kind of eventuality was unsuccessful in preventing the global spread of the disease.

Failures of intelligence and warning cannot explain the full story of the COVID-19 crisis, of course; many other failures and missteps have contributed to making the pandemic the catastrophe it has been. It seems clear that for many reasons the coronavirus was likely to have become a global pandemic no matter what we could have done. But the tragedy could have been significantly reduced through better warning mechanisms and with more attention paid to those warnings; and efforts to improve our global intelligence and warning systems will be needed to anticipate and prevent another disaster next time.

The formal US intelligence community plays an important role in analyzing and warning of biological, medical, and other health threats—in particular, in dealing with biological warfare and terrorism but also with naturally caused threats such as infectious disease. The IC is not, however, the organization charged with the primary responsibility for collecting and analyzing intelligence on the threat of a pandemic. Within the US federal government, the Centers for Disease Control (CDC) has the lead on such efforts, but the US system of federalism grants states the primary responsibility for collecting public health data, which makes it difficult to monitor the course of an outbreak at the national level. Making it even more difficult is the larger job of collecting and analyzing global intelligence on viral threats, which belongs primarily to a network of national and international medical surveillance systems coordinated by the World Health Organization (WHO) through its efforts to validate disease reports and distribute early warning alerts.

Health experts as well as intelligence organizations have been warning for years about the threat of a global pandemic, but in the end these surveillance and warning systems were not enough to prevent disaster. How was it possible for the coronavirus to become so widespread and so deadly despite these warnings? There are many ways to answer this question, of course, and there were failings at many levels. Understanding how intelligence warnings work—or do not work—can help us understand why the years of warnings were not enough.

The failure of warning in the case of COVID-19 can be best understood by comparison with similar failures of warning preceding earlier catastrophes such as the 9/11 attacks and the attack on Pearl Harbor, which I have examined in other works.[12] The use of intelligence to prevent surprise attacks suggests that long-term strategic warning, of the sort we saw in the years before the coronavirus pandemic began, is almost completely ineffective in preventing surprise and disaster. These big-picture warnings of possible threats to come tend to have very little impact on leaders who are preoccupied with problems and challenges they face today. This is what happened when the United States was surprised both at Pearl Harbor and on 9/11, as years of strategic warnings had little impact on the decision-makers and failed to prevent surprise and disaster. This happened again in early 2020, when the United States and the world were surprised by what was essentially a surprise attack by a deadly virus.

Two factors are needed to make intelligence actionable and disaster preventable: *specific tactical-level warning* and *receptive decision-makers*. Tactical-level intelligence must be collected and conveyed to decision-makers in near real time as a threat arises, and decision-makers must have the training and experience with intelligence to be receptive to the warnings they receive and take action as necessary. In the case of the coronavirus crisis, neither of these factors was available to the level that allowed the threat to be sufficiently contained. A key problem in the United States and abroad was a lack of clear, precise intelligence and warning during the critical early weeks and months of the pandemic, when action could have been most effective. Even when warning was available, too often leaders failed to pay attention.

From what we now know, the coronavirus crisis did not display the level of intelligence failure and mismanagement seen before the 9/11 attacks. For example, unlike in the 9/11 case where intelligence agencies had information on future hijackers that they failed to share with other agencies, it appears that the US intelligence community responded appropriately—if ultimately insufficiently—as early indications of the new virus began to appear. At the same time, however, the coronavirus pandemic does demonstrate many of the same problems related to intelligence that were seen on 9/11, such as the failure of the George W. Bush administration to take action before the attacks despite having received multiple warnings about the threat posed by Osama bin Laden and al Qaeda.

Similarly, before the coronavirus pandemic the Trump administration took a number of steps that reduced the nation's ability to respond quickly to a major public health emergency, including eliminating the office within the NSC that focused on global health security.[13] We know that President Trump was aware of the severity of the COVID-19 threat as early as February 7, 2020, when he told journalist Bob Woodward that the virus was more dangerous than the flu yet declined to take decisive action.[14]

Trump's failure to act will likely rank as one of the most notable cases in which politically motivated behavior and neglect of intelligence led to calamity.[15] But this is not a book about Donald Trump. Although he and his administration played a leading role in the story of how America responded (or failed to respond) to the coronavirus, the story is much bigger than any one president, any one administration, or any one country. Trump's disregard for the threat does not fully explain the lack of early, decisive actions to stem the outbreak in the United States—where many of the most important public health decisions and actions are taken on a state or local basis—or in many countries around the world. That lack of action can be largely explained by the ineffectiveness of strategic warning, the failure of tactical-level intelligence, and the absence of receptive decision-makers.

The COVID-19 pandemic must serve as a wake-up call for the United States and the international community; it demonstrates that we live in an era in which threats from infectious disease are much more dangerous than ever before. Actionable intelligence can be developed on future pandemic and health threats and leaders can become receptive to the warnings they receive. But a global effort will be needed if we are to develop the intelligence systems and capabilities that will anticipate and prevent the next crisis.

## THE PLAN OF THE BOOK

Chapter 1 asks whether infectious diseases and pandemics should be considered a national security problem and, if so, what that means for policy. Should pandemics be addressed using traditional national security methods and organizations, including intelligence agencies? Or would it be better to let those agencies focus on traditional security threats while governments and health organizations use public health tools such as disease surveillance to combat pandemics? It includes a review of the arguments of critics who believe health threats should not be considered as national security problems because they securitize or even militarize what should be treated as a public health issue, as well as those of national security experts who believe we should seize the moment of a pandemic to treat disease as a critical security threat.

Despite debates about the appropriateness of using national security tools to combat disease, the US intelligence community has for decades played a key role in warning about the risk of public health threats, including pandemics. Chapter 2 examines those responsibilities, including both the long-term strategic warning functions performed by top-level agencies, such as the Office of the Director of National Intelligence and the Central Intelligence Agency, and the more immediate alerting and reporting functions carried out by lesser-known organizations like the National Center for Medical Intelligence. The chapter also briefly discusses the basic concepts of intelligence and warning and reviews how intelligence-collection tools and disciplines can be used to combat health threats.

As important as the efforts of traditional national security intelligence agencies are, the primary task of detecting and warning of disease outbreaks belongs to a complex network of national and international medical intelligence and surveillance systems. Chapter 3 examines these systems, including the US medical surveillance efforts coordinated by the Centers for Disease Control as well as international programs, many of which fall under the World

Health Organization. It also discusses newer tools being used for disease surveillance, including artificial intelligence systems that scan global media, internet, and social media sites.

Chapter 4 reviews the performance of all of these organizations and systems—both traditional national security intelligence and medical and public
health systems—in the case of the COVID-19 pandemic. The chapter develops
the key argument of this book, which is that the pandemic was a global intelligence
failure—a failure remarkably similar to past failures of intelligence and warning,
such as Pearl Harbor and the 9/11 attacks. The comparison with 9/11 is especially instructive as we struggle today to understand how the pandemic occurred
despite the multiyear warnings by intelligence agencies and public health officials about just such a threat. The chapter explains how these strategic-level big-
picture warnings were not enough to inspire leaders to take action, while the kind
of intelligence that might have been effective—specific, tactical-level intelligence
in the early days and weeks of the outbreak—was tragically limited. Just as was
the case before the 9/11 attacks, US leaders—and leaders in many other countries
around the world—were unreceptive to the warnings they did receive.

As terrible as the coronavirus pandemic has been (and continues to be as
of this writing), the next global health threat could be even worse. Chapter 5
examines what the United States and the rest of the world must do to anticipate and prepare for the next pandemic. Major reforms are needed in the US
national security intelligence system, but even more important are changes
needed in our national and international medical and public health surveillance warning systems. Most urgent is the development of a global early warning system for infectious diseases and other health threats, but changes are
also needed at the national, state, and local levels. Even more broadly, we must
establish closer ties between the traditional intelligence, medical, and public
health communities.

The book's conclusion suggests that the lessons learned for intelligence
and warning from the coronavirus pandemic will not only be critical as we
prepare for the next pandemic; they are also important as we face other kinds
of threats in the future. The next great global disaster could arise from climate
change or some other natural disaster, from cyber threats, or in the form of a
global crisis fueled by natural as well as human-caused factors such as from
mass migration. It could develop out of a more conventional security crisis,
such as from rising tensions among the world's great powers, or it could come
from literally out of this world in the form of a megadisaster involving a solar
storm or asteroid impact. Regardless of the cause, global and national intelligence and warning systems will be needed to anticipate, detect, and respond
to those threats.

# NOTES

1. Langmuir, "The Surveillance of Communicable Diseases."
2. As of this writing the coronavirus pandemic has killed more than nine hundred thousand in the United States and over six million worldwide.
3. The formal name for the virus that created the current global pandemic is severe acute respiratory syndrome coronavirus 2, or SARS-CoV-2; the disease caused by this virus is coronavirus disease 2019, or COVID-19. This book refers to "coronavirus" and COVID-19 interchangeably.
4. James B. Rule and Han Cheng, "Coronavirus and the Surveillance State," *Dissent*, Summer 2020, https://www.dissentmagazine.org/article/coronavirus-and-the-surveillance -state.
5. Laqueur, "The Question of Judgment," 534.
6. David Omand, "Will the Intelligence Agencies Spot the Next Outbreak?," *The Article*, May 18, 2020, https://www.thearticle.com/will-the-intelligence-agencies-spot -the-next-outbreak.
7. Calder Walton, "US Intelligence, the Coronavirus and the Age of Globalized Challenges," Centre for International Governance Innovation, August 24, 2020, https:// www.cigionline.org/articles/us-intelligence-coronavirus-and-age-globalized -challenges.
8. Bernard, "Health and National Security," 158.
9. Tara O'Toole and Margaret Bourdeaux, "Intelligence Failure? How Divisions Between Intelligence and Public Health Left Us Vulnerable to a Pandemic," Belfer Center for Science and International Affairs, https://www.belfercenter.org/event /intelligence-failure-how-divisions-between-intelligence-and-public-health-left -us-vulnerable.
10. On the lack of knowledge, see Harley Feldbaum, "US Global Health and National Security Policy," Center for Strategic and International Studies, April 20, 2009, 2, https://www.csis.org/analysis/us-global-health-and-national-security-policy. On disseminating information, see Cecchine and Moore, "Infectious Disease and National Security."
11. Osterholm and Olshaker, "Chronicle of a Pandemic Foretold," 13.
12. Dahl, *Intelligence and Surprise Attack.*
13. Lena H. Sun, "Top White House Official in Charge of Pandemic Response Exits Abruptly," *Washington Post*, May 10, 2018, https://www.washingtonpost.com /news/to-your-health/wp/2018/05/10/top-white-house-official-in-charge-of -pandemic-response-exits-abruptly/.
14. Maggie Haberman, "Trump Admits Downplaying the Virus Knowing It Was 'Deadly Stuff,'" *New York Times*, September 9, 2020, https://www.nytimes.com /2020/09/09/us/politics/woodward-trump-book-virus.html.
15. For other examples, see Bar-Joseph and Levy, "Conscious Action and Intelligence Failure"; and Bar-Joseph and McDermott, *Intelligence Success and Failure.*

# ONE

# Are Pandemics a National Security Problem?

In the wake of the COVID-19 pandemic it might seem unnecessary or even foolish to ask whether an infectious disease or other health issue should be considered a national security problem. The answer might simply be: of course it should! After all, COVID-19 killed millions worldwide and created what may be the greatest economic crisis in the United States since the Great Depression, and world leaders have often used the language of war to describe the struggle against it.[1] The United States and many other nations mobilized military forces to combat the virus and, among the many other obvious national security effects, the fallout from the pandemic forced a US aircraft carrier to shore and led to the resignation of the secretary of the navy.

But is the language of war an appropriate way to describe a pandemic or other health threat? Critics argue that it merely securitizes and even militarizes what should instead be treated as a public health problem.[2] Should disease be considered a matter of national security, addressed using traditional security means (including intelligence agencies), or would it be better to let those agencies focus on traditional security threats while governments respond to pandemic threats through medical and public health efforts and by increasing support for organizations such as the Centers for Disease Control (CDC) and the World Health Organization (WHO)? If we do consider infectious disease to be a national security problem, what does that mean?

I argue that pandemics and other health threats are indeed a national security problem and that it is appropriate to consider them so. They are national security issues not only because of their potentially grave health impacts and the effect they can have on traditional security areas, but also because, as we have seen with COVID-19 and previous outbreaks, health disasters have tremendous impact in social, economic, and political areas as well. This chapter first examines the use of the "war" metaphor, followed by a review of the arguments of those who believe pandemics and other health threats should *not* be considered national security problems and how the US national security establishment has dealt with such threats. The final section takes a more theoretical approach to develop an argument for why pandemics and other health threats should indeed be considered a national security problem.

## WAR FOOTING OR DANGEROUS SECURITIZATION?

Leaders around the world have readily used the language of war in discussing the COVID-19 pandemic. In China, President Xi Jinping declared a "people's war"; in France, President Emmanuel Macron put the country on a "war footing"; in the United States, Donald Trump called himself a "war-time president."[3] Many experts, including former and current US national security leaders, have argued the pandemic shows that health must be considered a national security issue. Samantha Power, ambassador to the United Nations (UN) under President Barack Obama and administrator of the US Agency for International Development (USAID) under President Joe Biden, wrote that "the shared enemy of a future pandemic must bring about a redefinition of national security and generate long overdue increases of federal investments in domestic and global health security preparedness."[4] Michele Flournoy, former undersecretary of defense, has said that threats like COVID-19 "should be part of our national security thinking and rubric."[5] Yale Law School professor Oona Hathaway put it this way: "If one believes, as I do, that the fundamental goal of a national security program should be to protect American lives, then we clearly have our priorities out of place. Just as the 9/11 attacks led to a reorientation of national security policy around a counterterrorism mission, the COVID-19 crisis can and should lead to a reorientation of national security policy."[6]

On the other hand, critics of that type of thinking warn that we should not treat a pandemic—which is essentially a public health problem—as we would a military or national security threat.[7] That is, using the language of war is inappropriate and could lead to the use of military and national intelligence tools in ways that are counterproductive, much as many argue that law enforcement in the United States after the 9/11 terrorist attacks became militarized and led to overreaction and an unnecessary use of force when police responded to protests after the death of George Floyd. Lawrence Freedman points out that people who declare "wars" against enemies such as inflation rarely end up winning: "When governments use war analogies to respond to national emergencies they invite disappointment."[8]

Christine Schwöbel-Patel notes that "we tend to forget that emergency powers have a habit of sticking around far longer than the crisis requires."[9] The use of a war metaphor, she argues, encourages talk of an "enemy," which builds nationalist sentiment rather than the coordination and cooperation needed. Other critics warn that history shows that when governments adopt warlike measures to deal with threats—such as after 9/11—the result is often restrictions on civil liberties and expansion of government power that remain in effect far longer than was initially envisioned.[10]

Catherine Connolly writes: "The use of the war metaphor and the language of violence and conflict is neither accurate nor helpful for the situation we are facing. For one thing, those drawing parallels between this pandemic and war fail to recognise the role of war in spreading disease, and in causing public health crises. The relationship between war and disease is not benign, and it is certainly not positive—war does not cure or cleanse."[11] Catherine Lutz and Neta Crawford make a similar point, arguing that "war" is the wrong metaphor for the struggle against COVID-19 and military bellicosity is the wrong context. Instead of militarized solutions, they argue, we need civilian solutions for the problems of health and disease.[12] Former assistant secretary of defense Sharon Burke writes that we need a different vision of security, because our current focus on hard power has actually made us weaker: "The pandemic has underscored the truth that the United States needs to redefine security to include everything that makes us safe, from cooperative global relationships to a healthy ecosystem."[13]

There is little doubt that infectious disease is a threat to *human* security. As noted by Ronald Klain, Obama's Ebola response coordinator in 2014–15 and Biden's chief of staff, infectious diseases have "killed more humans that all wars, terrorist attacks, and natural disasters *combined.*"[14] Other experts have made similar points. Andrew Price-Smith, for example, writes that "throughout recorded history, infectious disease has consistently accounted for the greatest proportion of human morbidity and mortality, surpassing war as the foremost threat to human life and prosperity."[15] Furthermore, there is a clear link between health and traditional security issues such as war; for example, scholars have examined the relationship between health and conflict and have found that disease and other health problems tend to produce instability.[16]

Does this mean that disease and health threats should be considered a matter of national security? As Susan Peterson writes, "Health issues have not permeated the national security field, which traditionally has focused on the preservation of the state from physical threats."[17] If we do consider infectious disease to be a national security problem, what does that mean and why might it matter?

As Dexter Fergie has described, the use of the term "national security" is a relatively recent phenomenon in US history, only becoming common during and after World War II. Before then it was more common for military and civilian leaders to talk about "national defense," and out of that context only more narrowly discussing matters of war and peace. More recently, "national security" has been used by leaders to describe a wide variety of problems and challenges, so much so that, as Fergie puts it, "now, 'national security' threatens to swallow everything."[18]

As Peterson notes, there have been periods during which security studies scholars and experts have pressed for a broader understanding of security to include health and disease, such as during the HIV/AIDS epidemic and following 9/11, amid concerns of biological terrorism.[19] Scholars and practitioners who focus on human security are more likely to view infectious disease as a threat to security.[20] But, as treatments have been developed for HIV/AIDS and early dire predictions about bioterror have not come to pass, the interest in making the health-security link has declined.[21] Traditional security studies scholars have often argued against expanding the definition of security beyond a focus on physical threats to the state. Daniel Deudney, for example, writes about linking environmental issues with security: "Not all threats to life and property are threats to security. Disease, old age, crime and accidents routinely destroy life and property, but we do not think of them as 'national security' threats or even threats to 'security.'"[22]

## The Problem of Securitization

A number of scholars have used securitization theory, as developed by the Copenhagen school of international relations, as a model for understanding how health can be viewed as a security issue.[23] "Securitization" is a process by which a political or any issue is framed as a security problem, which enables the use of extraordinary measures such as military force.[24] Securitization can have the advantage of helping focus attention and resources on a particular disease. Thomas Abraham, for example, has argued that the H1N1 influenza outbreak in 2009 received the global attention it did only because the United States took the lead on securitizing the threat, lifting if from the public health arena to the realm of national and global security.[25] But, as Stefan Elbe points out regarding the case of the outbreak of H5N1 avian flu in 2005–6, securitization can also have the unwanted effect of politicizing a disease and delaying or obstructing potential responses due to political or diplomatic disputes.[26]

Paul Rogers has written about this danger in the context of COVID-19, warning about the dangers of "securitizing the pandemic as a threat to be controlled, not a common problem to be addressed cooperatively with an emphasis on aid to the weakest and most marginalized."[27] Rogers notes that in many countries a pandemic could exacerbate trends toward anti-immigration sentiment. A pandemic also could be seen as a threat to the more secure sectors of society, leading to increased suppression of protest and maintenance of security rather than on providing assistance to those in need. He also worries that securitization of a pandemic encourages the same thinking about climate change.

Other critics warn that securitization of infectious diseases "is not motivated by global health promotion but by the narrow security interest of developed countries."[28] As Simon Rushton has described this view, "The developing world is being asked to bear many of the costs of ensuring global health security, but suspicions are evident in some quarters that these measures may in fact be primarily about the protections of the West."[29] Rushton further states it more bluntly: "It is no wonder that some fear that the real agenda behind the promotion of the concept of global health security . . . is to protect the developed world from diseases that, epidemiologically speaking, tend to emerge from the developing world."[30]

Debra L. DeLaet writes that securitization can help focus attention and attract funding for diseases, such as was done successfully with HIV/AIDS. But she notes that health securitization also tends to encourage state-focused policies that rely on traditional security institutions and programs at the expense of public health actors and broader health initiatives that address more fundamental health threats, such as those associated with poverty.[31] Yanzhong Huang makes a similar point, noting that securitization can encourage the use of traditional military measures such as quarantine as opposed to an increase in capacity for efforts against the disease and to encourage whole of society and international cooperation.[32]

As one critic has written, focusing on health security too often focuses on emerging infectious diseases to the neglect of broader threats to human security:

> An alternative approach to health security would recognise that the broader determinants of health does not simply mean replacing "bombs and bullets" with nasty pathogens. It begins with an understanding of how human health is intimately connected with the health of the planet, and then with the health of the social environments in which we live. Invariably, this requires us to take a global perspective because so many health determinants are not confined to state boundaries.[33]

Colin McInnes and Anne Roemer-Mahler argue that framing global health issues as risks, rather than as security issues, is less politically charged and divisive.[34] Peterson argues that considering health as a national security threat will actually be counterproductive, in that it will lead to states reinforcing national boundaries and becoming even less likely to cooperate with other states on health issues.[35] She also argues that encouraging international efforts against disease based only on narrow national security grounds may lead the West to act in its own narrow self-interest, relieving it of the moral obligation to help developing nations.

Harley Feldbaum and his colleagues argue that "treating global health issues as national security threats may focus attention disproportionately on countries or diseases which pose security threats to wealthy nations, rather than on the greatest threats to global health."[36] If care is not taken, they warn, "there is a risk that global health will be reduced to a bit player on the grand stage of power politics."[37]

Alexandre Christoyannopoulos argues that war metaphors mislead, because they bring to mind the use of military weapons and killing and they encourage national, state-based responses and minimize the role of international organizations and other actors. The use of such metaphors can also serve to "normalize war," encouraging us to turn to military solutions the next time. Christoyannopoulos cautions that "the coronavirus crisis is an international, pan-human challenge. It certainly requires exceptional collective mobilisation, but no real weapons, no intentional killing of fellow human beings, and no casting of people as dehumanised others. Militarised language is unnecessary."[38] Other experts such as Christian Enemark argue that the most important approach to epidemic disease control is through international cooperation so adopting a narrow national security focus could work against that goal.[39]

Some public health experts have in fact suggested that the language and the logic should be the other way around: rather than considering whether disease and health should be considered as problems akin to war, we should consider whether war is a public health problem.[40] Surveillance studies scholars such as Martin French argue that public health surveillance in the United States has become militarized, using the language of war and defending the body against enemies. This tends to nationalize and even globalize disease surveillance for the benefit of the powerful, and marginalize the needs and concerns of the individual.[41] Stefan Elbe argues that it can be useful for public health professionals to "play the security card" when it comes to the threat of bioterrorism and biological warfare, as this can help make resources available and get the attention of leaders.[42]

More generally, the professional cultures of public health and national security are so different that some in the health field believe they risk losing their objectivity and independence if they are seen as coordinating with the security community. Elbe cautions that "'security' is a politically deeply charged and sensitive notion—the pursuit of which has in the past enabled states to override legal constraints and justify a range of extraordinary and also controversial practices."[43] While a human security approach may be the right way to bring together health and security, the greatest concern is not infectious diseases or deliberate bio attacks but rather the range of illnesses that affect people around the world, such as malaria, TB, and AIDS.

The blurry lines between health and security were demonstrated in the US military and intelligence effort to find and ultimately kill Osama bin Laden in 2011. Part of that effort involved creating a fake Hepatitis B vaccination campaign in Abbottabad, Pakistan, in order to detect the presence of bin Laden family DNA in the compound where the al Qaeda leader was suspected to be hiding. The immunizations offered were real, but public health officials have raised the concern that the revelations about the program risked reducing future trust in public health measures in Pakistan and elsewhere.[44]

## HEALTH SECURITY IN THE US NATIONAL SECURITY ESTABLISHMENT

US leaders have been calling for a broader definition of national security for some time. What may have been the first formal US government acknowledgment of disease as a national security threat came in 1996, with President Clinton's Presidential Decision Directive NSTC-7, which declared: "Emerging infectious diseases . . . present one of the most significant health challenges facing the global community."[45] In a speech to the National Council for International Health marking the rollout of the new policy established in that presidential directive, Vice President Al Gore said, "Today, guaranteeing national security means more than just defending our borders at home and our values abroad or having the best-trained armed forces in the world. Now it also means defending our nation's health against all enemies, foreign and domestic."[46]

The traditional elements of the US national security establishment have long considered health to be a significant security issue. In 1997, for example, the US Department of Defense (DoD) formed the Global Emerging Infections Surveillance and Response System (GEIS) in order to watch for emerging diseases that could affect the US military.[47] Additionally, the US intelligence community has for decades considered infectious diseases to be a national security threat, marked by a National Intelligence Estimate published in January 2000. That estimate stated that "new and reemerging infectious diseases will pose a rising global health threat and will complicate US and global security over the next 20 years. These diseases will endanger US citizens at home and abroad, threaten US armed forces deployed overseas, and exacerbate social and political instability in key countries and regions in which the United States has significant interests."[48]

Concerns about the threat of bioterrorism, and calls for surveillance efforts to counter that threat, began to be heard in the late 1990s.[49] Then after the 9/11 attacks, and especially as a response to the anthrax attacks that followed shortly after 9/11, leaders such as President Bush used the language of national security in calling for greater efforts to combat the threat of bioterrorism. In 2002 Bush visited the University of Pittsburgh Medical Center and praised the Real Time Outbreak and Disease Surveillance Project, which was designed to gather information from area hospitals so that suspicious cases could be quickly identified. Bush likened the system to the DEW Line of the early Cold War that was designed to warn of enemy bombers flying over the North Pole, saying, "Well, here in Pittsburgh, I had the honor of seeing a demonstration of the modern DEW Line, a real-time outbreak and disease-surveillance system developed right here, which is one of the country's leading centers on monitoring biological threats."[50]

Scholars such as Andrew Price-Smith have noted that this post-9/11 emphasis on bioterrorism has neglected broader aspects of public health and in particular global health concerns.[51] Although bioterrorism has certainly been a key concern for US defense and national security officials, naturally occurring disease threats continue to be identified as national security concerns, such as in reports from think tanks and blue-ribbon commissions.[52] The Project on National Security Reform proposed in 2008 "a new concept of national security" that included the need "to maintain security against massive societal disruption as a result of natural forces, including pandemics, natural disasters, and climate change."[53]

The concern about health security continued through the Obama administration. Obama's 2010 National Security Strategy defined security broadly, arguing that threats to US security had evolved to include economic instability, environmental damage, food insecurity, and dangers to public health.[54] President Obama spoke to the UN General Assembly in 2011 and called upon all countries to come together to combat biological dangers ranging from pandemics to terrorist attacks.[55] Health threats were also seen as significant homeland security threats; the Department of Homeland Security, for example, in 2014 declared that "biological threats and hazards—ranging from bioterrorism to naturally occurring pandemics—are a top homeland security risk."[56]

Under President Trump, however, the focus shifted back to more conventional threats, including especially a concern about great-power competition. The Trump administration's 2017 National Security Strategy, for example, acknowledged that "biological threats to the U.S. homeland—whether as the result of deliberate attack, accident, or a natural outbreak—are growing and require actions to address them at their source."[57] But the document placed greater emphasis on traditional national security concerns: border security, counterterrorism, and competition with China and Russia.

Since the outbreak of the COVID-19 pandemic, numerous national security experts have argued the United States needs to seize the moment and acknowledge that disease should be treated like a critical national security threat. As one expert told the *Washington Post*, "We need to treat this moment like we treated 9/11, recognizing that we have a massive vulnerability in which we have chronically underinvested."[58] Dr. Julie Gerberding, co-chair of the CSIS Commission on Strengthening America's Health Security, testified in June 2020, "We began the Commission's work with a simple understanding: health security is national security, in a world that is increasingly dangerous and interdependent."[59] Lisa Monaco, Obama's advisor for homeland security and counterterrorism, argues in *Foreign Affairs* that "the time is long past to make pandemic disease a national security priority commensurate with the threat it poses to global security and stability."[60]

### Health as a Security Concern beyond the United States

Health issues have often been described as security concerns by other countries and the international community, dating back to at least 2000, when the UN Security Council for the first time designated a disease, HIV/AIDS, as a threat to international security.[61] In a speech to the Security Council Gore argued that infectious disease such as AIDS need to be included in a "new, more expansive definition" of security, while UN Secretary-General Kofi Annan said the impact of AIDS in Africa "was no less destructive than that of warfare itself."[62]

The United Kingdom is an example of a country that has a track record of viewing health and pandemics as a national security concern. It regularly publishes a National Risk Register that outlines the most significant threats facing the UK population. In 2010 the register ranked the risk of pandemic disease as the highest, writing what appears prescient today: "In addition to the severe health effects, a pandemic is also likely to cause significant wider social and economic damage and disruption."[63] The UK Ministry of Defence has also seen infectious disease as a threat to national security, such as in its Global Strategic Trends series. The series' latest report, published in 2018 and released before the COVID-19 outbreak, noted in what might today seem like British understatement: "Although we are currently better at fighting infectious disease than at any other time in history, the risk of a global pandemic could be increasing."[64]

## A MORE THEORETICAL ARGUMENT

Ever since Thucydides described the plague that devastated Athens during the Peloponnesian War in the fifth century BCE, historians and scholars from many different communities have long noted the close connection between war and public health.[65] A century after the Spanish flu of 1918 killed more people than World War I itself, many military, intelligence, and other national security organizations have treated disease as a security issue. It may be, as Simon Rushton has written, that "the securitization ship has already sailed."[66]

But other experts have argued that treating health and disease as a national security problem can be counterproductive and lead to the use of inappropriate tools that support the interests of wealthier nations at the expense of poorer and weaker ones.

How, then, can we decide whether disease and health should be considered national security problems? We can find the answer by first asking what we mean by "national security" and then determining whether disease and health threats fit that definition.

Although there is no clear agreement among experts on what constitutes "national security," there has been a noticeable shift in the use of the term since the early Cold War, from the narrow to the broad. As Helga Haftendorn has described, in the decades following World War II the focus was on the narrow military sense of the term, with national survival seen as the prime goal of national security.[67] By the 1980s, however, experts had come to recognize that purely military approaches were insufficient. In a widely cited 1983 article, Richard Ullman argued for a broader definition of national security beyond military concerns, to include threats that might degrade the quality of life or reduce the range of policy options available to leaders and citizens.[68] A few years later, in an article with the same title as Ullman's, Jessica Tuchman Mathews made a similar argument, writing that the concept of national security needed to be broadened again, to include resource and environmental concerns and demographic issues.[69]

When President George W. Bush came into office in February 2001, his first National Security Presidential Directive defined the term this way: "National security includes the defense of the United States of America, protection of our constitutional system of government, and the advancement of United States interests around the globe. National security also depends on America's opportunity to prosper in the world economy."[70] In 2008 the Project on National Security Reform argued for an even broader definition, to include not only defending the nation from external aggression, but also from threats that could cause "massive societal disruption" or could lead to failure of major national infrastructure systems.[71]

Clearly the COVID-19 pandemic has created massive societal disruption across the globe, but is that sufficient cause for declaring it a national security issue and employing the tools of national security to deal with it? One can imagine other problems and forces that might disrupt society but which need not be considered national security problems. To avoid overcompensating, we might argue that disease and health issues—and presumably other kinds of nontraditional threats—can be considered national security problems only if they have a significant impact on the military or other aspects of traditional security.

From this vantage point—through its effect on US and other military forces—the COVID-19 pandemic can clearly be seen as a national security issue. The United States withdrew from bases in Iraq, NATO suspended training, and an exercise called Defender-20, the largest movement of US troops to Europe since the Cold War, was halted and then scaled back after one Polish general involved in the exercise became sick.[72] The greatest impact may have been on navies, including forcing the USS *Theodore Roosevelt* to halt operations and return to port in Guam, while France's only aircraft carrier, the *Charles De Gaulle*, was also taken out of action after two-thirds of its crew became infected.[73] As two security experts put it, "For the first time since World War II, an adversary managed to knock a U.S. Navy aircraft carrier out of service."[74]

This relatively narrow definition of when disease becomes a national security issue is similar to the argument made by Peterson, who writes, "The heart of the link between [infectious diseases] and national security concerns the effect of catastrophic disease on violent conflict."[75] By this way of thinking, disease threatens national security either by contributing to the outbreak of or influencing the outcome of violent conflict. It is tempting to adopt this definition, because we have many examples through history of how war and disease are related. That link is occasionally very clear, such as when armies have use biological weapons against opposing forces as well as civilians.[76] And the relationship between conflict and disease can work both ways, as war can worsen the spread of disease but disease can also, according to many experts, increase the likelihood and severity of war. As *The Economist* put it, "War and disease feed upon each other."[77]

There is debate among scholars, however, on whether disease does actually tend to amplify or increase the chance of war. Some experts have argued that while disease and pandemics can make states more aggressive in the short run, in the long run disease tends to weaken states and reduce their ability to project military power.[78] Andrew Price-Smith, one of the most insightful thinkers on the relationship between disease and conflict, writes that "there is considerable weight to the proposition that war acts to amplify disease, but there is little current empirical evidence to support the hypothesis that disease fosters war between sovereign states."[79] Although we can acknowledge a long history of war and disease accompanying each other, Price-Smith argues that the relationship may actually be a form of negative feedback loop: conflict initially amplifies disease, but ultimately the spread of infection within military units may reduce their ability to conduct operations and lead to a decrease in bellicosity.[80]

Price-Smith argues that only diseases that threaten national security through lethality, economic damage, or other effects should be considered security threats. Some diseases, such as Lyme disease, are treatable and not likely to be a security threat. Others, such as measles, affect primarily the very young and very old, so although they could be considered human security concerns, they are not likely to have a significant impact on military forces and thus do not represent a threat to national security.[81] With these considerations in mind, Price-Smith develops a set of criteria to evaluate whether a given pathogen constitutes a security threat:

- Results in a minimum 1 percent reduction in GDP
- Kills 1 percent of the total adult population per year
- Severely debilitates 10 percent of the total adult population per year[82]

Such criteria are controversial, and Price-Smith acknowledges that his intent in proposing them was to stimulate debate. It seems that his definition of national security is too narrow, and the experience of the COVID-19 pandemic has taught us that infectious disease can impact national and international security in many ways beyond reducing military capabilities or reaching specific benchmarks.

Other experts have suggested using different benchmarks to determine whether a public health threat should be considered a national security threat. James Hodge and Kim Weidenaar offer these ten criteria:

- Threatens political or social stability
- Reduces the ability of vulnerable groups in society to participate in that society
- Imperils domestic or international economic stability
- Has the potential to weaken or diminish military power, whether through the spread of infectious disease or through the impact of other health conditions (such as the problem of obesity among young adults)
- Produces impacts that cross national borders
- Arises from nonstate actors, such as when the overuse of antibiotics by healthcare providers produces antibiotic-resistant bacteria
- Exceeds the ability of national health systems to control it
- Creates the potential for systematic human rights abuses
- Is beyond global public health systems' response capabilities
- Encourages leaders to classify it as a national security concern due to public perceptions[83]

This model has the advantage of being relatively comprehensive, but a simpler model is probably more useful for determining when a health threat—or some other nontraditional concern—merits being considered a threat to national security.

A threat becomes a national security issue when it meets two basic criteria:

- It has a significant impact on a wide variety of sectors in society, including not just the military and traditional national security but also the economic and social sectors.
- Societies must use a wide range of tools, including but not limited to the tools of the military and the national security apparatus to successfully address it.

Using this simple set of criteria, it is clear that pandemics and other health threats do indeed qualify as national security concerns. They are national security issues not only because of their potentially grave health impacts and the effects they can have on national security, but also because, as we have seen with COVID-19 and previous outbreaks, they have tremendous impacts on social, economic, and political areas. The struggle against these threats requires a whole-of-society effort, including the military and other national security institutions. However, viewing a pandemic as a national security concern does not mean the military should be in charge of the response. To put it another way, "securitization" in the context of COVID-19 does not equate to "militarization."

Although the current focus is on the threat produced by disease and other health issues, we should note that the debate over whether health issues, including COVID-19, should be considered threats to national security is similar in some ways to the debate over whether other transnational issues, such as climate change, are also significant threats. Scholars such as Price-Smith have often noted the similarity between discussions about health security and environmental security, and this proposed model can be useful in examining the national security implications of other nontraditional threats as well.

## CONCLUSION

Disease and health threats such as the COVID-19 pandemic should indeed be considered national security threats. This question of definition is more than an academic matter, because defining infectious disease as a national security threat means that in addition to using the tools of medicine and public health, we should be prepared to bring to bear tools that are more typically used against traditional security threats. Some of these most important tools are those of intelligence, surveillance, and warning, which are indeed the purview of the US intelligence community.

# NOTES

1. Lawrence Freedman, "Coronavirus and the Language of War," *New Statesman*, April 11, 2020, https://www.newstatesman.com/science-tech/2020/04/coronavirus-and-language-war.
2. For an example, see Alexandre Christoyannopoulos, "Stop Calling Coronavirus Pandemic a 'War,'" *The Conversation*, April 7, 2020, https://theconversation.com/stop-calling-coronavirus-pandemic-a-war-135486; and Alex de Waal, "Militarizing Global Health," *Boston Review*, November 11, 2014, https://bostonreview.net/world/alex-de-waal-militarizing-global-health-ebola.
3. Freedman, "Coronavirus and the Language of War."
4. Samantha Power, "How the COVID-19 Era Will Change National Security Forever," *Time*, April 14, 2020, https://time.com/5820625/national-security-coronavirus-samantha-power/.
5. Cited in Gronvall, "The Scientific Response to COVID-19," 83.
6. Oona Hathaway, "COVID-19 Shows How the U.S. Got National Security Wrong," *Just Security* (blog), April 7, 2020, https://www.justsecurity.org/69563/covid-19-shows-how-the-u-s-got-national-security-wrong/.
7. Christoyannopoulos, "Stop Calling Coronavirus." A succinct discussion of both sides of the issue is Enemark, "Is Pandemic Flu a Security Threat?." I should note that public health is a very large field covering many elements of human health. There are important debates about whether some issues, such as the prevalence of obesity, should be considered national security problems. But this book's focus is on the subset of public health issues that includes pathogens with the potential to create pandemics or otherwise cause security disruptions. I am grateful to an anonymous reviewer for this point.
8. Freedman, "Coronavirus and the Language of War."
9. Christine Schwöbel-Patel, "We Don't Need a 'War' against Coronavirus, We Need Solidarity," Aljazeera.com, April 6, 2020.
10. Indra Ekmanis, "How 'War' with Coronavirus Could Lead to Lasting Government Overreach," *The World*, March 19, 2020, https://www.pri.org/stories/2020-03-19/how-war-coronavirus-could-lead-lasting-government-overreach.
11. Catherine Connolly, "War and the Coronavirus Pandemic," *Third World Approaches to International Law Review*, April 9, 2020, https://twailr.com/war-and-the-coronavirus-pandemic/.
12. Catherine Lutz and Neta C. Crawford, "Fighting a Virus with the Wrong Tools," *The Hill*, March 28, 2020, https://thehill.com/opinion/finance/489733-fighting-a-virus-with-the-wrong-tools.
13. Sharon E. Burke, "US Security Requires Far More than a Strong Military," *Boston Globe*, July 15, 2020, https://www.bostonglobe.com/2020/07/15/opinion/us-security-requires-far-more-than-strong-military/.
14. Klain, "Confronting the Pandemic Threat" (emphasis in original).
15. Price-Smith, *The Health of Nations*, 2.
16. For a review of this literature, see Davies, "Healthy Populations."
17. Peterson, "Global Health and Security," 2.
18. Dexter Fergie, "The Strange Career of 'National Security,'" *Atlantic*, September 29, 2019. For a more extended discussion, see Fergie, "Geopolitics Turned Inwards."

19. Peterson, "Global Health and Security"; Peterson, "Epidemic Disease and National Security."
20. See, for example, Maclean, "Microbes, Mad Cows."
21. Peterson, "Global Health and Security."
22. Deudney, "The Case Against Linking," 463.
23. See, for example, Lo Yuk-ping and Thomas, "How Is Health a Security Issue?" See also Kamradt-Scott and McInnes, "The Securitisation of Pandemic Influenza."
24. Buzan, Waever, and de Wilde, *Security*.
25. Abraham, "The Chronicle of a Disease Foretold."
26. Elbe, "Haggling over Viruses." Useful overviews of the issues involved with the securitization of health are Baringer and Heitkamp, "Securitizing Global Health"; and Maclean, "Microbes, Mad Cows."
27. Paul Rogers, "COVID-19: The Dangers of Securitisation," *Oxford Research Group* (blog), September 29, 2020, https://www.oxfordresearchgroup.org.uk/covid-19 -the-dangers-of-securitisation.
28. Jin and Karackattu, "Infectious Diseases and Securitization," 185.
29. Rushton, "Global Health Security," 780.
30. Rushton, 793.
31. DeLaet, "Whose Interests?," 339.
32. Huang, "Pandemics and Security."
33. Lee, review of "The Health of Nations," 683.
34. McInnes and Roemer-Mahler, "From Security to Risk."
35. Peterson, "Global Health and Security."
36. Feldbaum et al., "Global Health and National Security," 192.
37. Feldbaum et al., 197.
38. Christoyannopoulos, "Stop Calling Coronavirus."
39. Enemark, "Is Pandemic Flu a Security Threat?"
40. Hagopian, "Why Isn't War Properly Framed?"
41. French, "Woven of War-Time Fabrics." Jin and Karackattu make a similar argument in "Infectious Diseases and Securitization."
42. Elbe, "Should Health Professionals Play?"
43. Elbe, 221.
44. Bowsher, Milner, and Sullivan, "Medical Intelligence"; Sara Reardon, "CIA's Fake Vaccination Drive Angers Public Health World," *Science*, July 13, 2011, https:// www.sciencemag.org/news/2011/07/cias-fake-vaccination-drive-angers-public -health-world. For background on the search for bin Laden, see Dahl, "Finding Bin Laden."
45. White House, "Presidential Decision Directive NSTC-7," 2. For background on the issue, see Fearnley, "Redesigning Syndromic Surveillance."
46. Gore, "Emerging Infections."
47. A useful overview of the DoD's health security efforts is Thomas R. Cullison and J. Stephen Morrison, "The U.S. Department of Defense's Role in Health Security: Current Capabilities and Recommendations for the Future," Center for Strategic and International Studies, June 2019, https://healthsecurity.csis.org/articles/the -u-s-department-of-defense-s-role-in-health-security-current-capabilities-and -recommendations-for-the-future/.
48. NIC, "The Global Infectious Disease Threat," 5.

49. Fairchild, Bayer, and Colgrove, *Searching Eyes*, 246–49.

50. Associated Press, "Bush Stumps for Bioterrorism Preparation," *Tulsa World*, February 6, 2002, LexisNexis Uni.

51. Price-Smith, *Contagion and Chaos*, 191.

52. Brower and Chalk, *The Global Threat*.

53. Project on National Security Reform, "Forging a New Shield," November 2008, v, http://0183896.netsolhost.com/site/wp-content/uploads/2011/12/pnsr_forging_a _new_shield_report.pdf.

54. White House, "National Security Strategy." See also Kathleen J. McInnis, "COVID-19: National Security and Defense Strategy," Congressional Research Service, April 30, 2020.

55. White House, "Remarks by President Obama in Address to the United Nations General Assembly," September 21, 2011, https://obamawhitehouse.archives.gov /the-press-office/2011/09/21/remarks-president-obama-address-united-nations -general-assembly.

56. DHS, "The 2014 Quadrennial Homeland Security Review," 46.

57. White House, "National Security Strategy," 9.

58. Jeremy Konyndyk, quoted in Shane Harris and Missy Ryan, "To Prepare for the Next Pandemic, the U.S. Needs to Change Its National Security Priorities, Experts Say," *Washington Post*, June 16, 2020, https://www.washingtonpost.com/national-security /to-prepare-for-the-next-pandemic-the-us-needs-to-change-its-national-security -priorities-experts-say/2020/06/16/b99807c0-aa9a-11ea-9063-e69bd6520940 _story.html.

59. Julie L. Gerberding, "COVID-19: Lessons Learned to Prepare for the Next Pandemic," U.S. Senate Committee on Health, Education, Labor and Pensions, June 23, 2020, https://www.help.senate.gov/imo/media/doc/Gerberding5.pdf.

60. Lisa Monaco, "Pandemic Disease Is a Threat to National Security: Washington Should Treat It Like One," *Foreign Affairs*, March 3, 2020, https://www.foreignaffairs .com/articles/2020-03-03/pandemic-disease-threat-national-security.

61. Peterson, "Epidemic Disease and National Security"; Elbe, "Should Health Professionals Play?."

62. Gore cited in Peterson, "Epidemic Disease and National Security," 43. Annan's comments cited in UN Press Release SC/6781, "Security Council Holds Debate on Impact of AIDS on Peace and Security in Africa," January 10, 2000, https://www.un .org/press/en/2000/20000110.sc6781.doc.html.

63. UK Government Cabinet Office, "National Risk Register of Civil Emergencies," London, 2010, 7, https://assets.publishing.service.gov.uk/government/uploads/system /uploads/attachment_data/file/211853/nationalriskregister-2010.pdf.

64. UK Ministry of Defence, "Global Strategic Trends," 61.

65. Levy and Sidel, *War and Public Health*; Sidel and Levy, "War, Terrorism, and Public Health."

66. Rushton, *Security and Public Health*, 2.

67. Haftendorn, "The Security Puzzle," 8.

68. Ullman, "Redefining Security."

69. Mathews, "Redefining Security."

70. White House, "National Security Presidential Directive-1, 2. For useful background, see Catherine Dale, Nina M. Serafino, and Pat Towell, "Organizing the

U.S. Government for National Security: Overview of the Interagency Reform Debates," Congressional Research Service, December 16, 2008.

71. Project on National Security Reform, "Forging a New Shield," 453–54.

72. "COVID-19 Raises the Risks of Violent Conflict," *The Economist*, June 18, 2020, https://www.economist.com/international/2020/06/18/covid-19-raises-the-risks-of-violent-conflict; Giovanna De Maio, "NATO's Response to COVID-19: Lessons for Resilience and Readiness," policy brief, Brookings Institution, October 2020, https://www.brookings.edu/wp-content/uploads/2020/10/FP_20201028_nato_covid_demaio-1.pdf.

73. "COVID-19 Raises the Risks."

74. Gregory D. Koblentz and Michael Hunzeker, "National Security in the Age of Pandemics," *Defense One*, April 3, 2020, https://www.defenseone.com/ideas/2020/04/national-security-age-pandemics/164365/.

75. Peterson, "Epidemic Disease and National Security," 54.

76. Koblentz, *Living Weapons*, 11–13.

77. "COVID-19 Raises the Risks."

78. Lazar Berman and Jennifer Tischler, "After the Calamity: Unexpected Effects of Epidemics on War," *Strategy Bridge*, July 30, 2020, https://thestrategybridge.org/the-bridge/2020/7/30/after-the-calamity-unexpected-effects-of-epidemics-on-war.

79. Price-Smith, *Contagion and Chaos*, 160.

80. Price-Smith, 201.

81. Price-Smith, 208.

82. Price-Smith, 206.

83. Hodge and Weidenaar, "Public Health Emergencies," 90–93.

TWO

# What Is the Role of the
# US Intelligence Community?

Although most people may have been unaware of the fact until the current crisis, the eighteen agencies that make up the US intelligence community have for many years played an important role in tracking health threats such as disease and biological terrorism and warning about the risk of public health issues, including pandemics.[1] This chapter reviews those agencies and their responsibilities, discussing both the long-term strategic warning functions performed by top-level agencies such as the Office of the Director of National Intelligence (ODNI) and the Central Intelligence Agency (CIA), and the more immediate alerting and reporting functions carried out by lesser-known organizations such as the National Center for Medical Intelligence (NCMI).

The chapter touches on the basic concepts of intelligence and warning, noting the important difference between strategic and tactical intelligence, and reviews the array of basic intelligence-collection tools and disciplines and the kinds of intelligence that organizations can provide about infectious diseases and other biological threats. Brief case studies reveal how the traditional intelligence community (IC) has performed during past disease outbreaks. Often these agencies have capabilities and information sources that are not available to the medical and public health communities, which allow them to provide assessments that can complement the information decision-makers get from other experts. For example, for many years the CIA has used both classified and unclassified data in reporting on the intelligence and national security implications of diseases around the world.[2] During the 2014 Ebola outbreak the National Geospatial-Intelligence Agency (NGA) created a public website that provided unclassified geospatial and mapping information to support nongovernmental organizations and others fighting the disease on the front lines in Africa.[3]

Intelligence insiders and scholars acknowledge that the IC has a role to play concerning disease and health, but they generally argue that this function is quite secondary to the primary role of tracking traditional national security threats. As noted intelligence expert Mark Lowenthal writes, "The intelligence task with respect to health is largely one of tracking patterns of infection," although intelligence officials do track the pronouncements and behavior of foreign governments.[4] Lowenthal adds that "the fact that much intelligence for health and environmental issues can be drawn from OSINT [open-source intelligence] tends also to make these less compelling issues for intelligence officers, who revert to their professional ethos that their job is to steal secrets."[5]

Former senior British intelligence official David Omand argues that "the assessment of disease outbreaks is not the business of the intelligence community," and most intelligence professionals would probably agree.[6] But I will show that the national security *implications* of a disease outbreak are indeed the business of intelligence agencies and thus may well require that intelligence agencies do get in the business of assessing the outbreaks themselves.

## INTELLIGENCE FUNDAMENTALS

To judge from the way intelligence professionals are portrayed in popular fiction, one might assume that the job of intelligence involves constant travel, adventure, and danger. But, unfortunately perhaps, the daily existence of most intelligence personnel is much more mundane; although some jobs certainly do involve travel and can even be exciting at times, intelligence collectors and analysts are much more likely to work behind a desk or at a computer than they are to be flying on private jets or staying at luxury hotels.

Although there are many possible ways to describe intelligence work, one of the most common among intelligence professionals is through what are known as the "ints," or the various disciplines of the intelligence business. These are the collection specialties through which intelligence agencies collect the raw information that makes up the ingredients of finished intelligence. Some of these specialties are widely recognized, such as human intelligence, or HUMINT, obtained through contact or communication with people. Human intelligence—also called espionage—has been described as the world's second oldest profession.[7] It is a core tool of intelligence agencies, and both openly gathered and clandestine (or secret) HUMINT can be of great use in detecting and analyzing disease threats.[8] The primary human intelligence organization in the United States is the Central Intelligence Agency (CIA), although other organizations also have important HUMINT missions; the Defense Intelligence Agency (DIA), for example, collects overt human intelligence through the reporting of military attaches posted overseas, as does the US State Department, from US diplomats stationed at locations around the world.

Signals intelligence (SIGINT) is another fundamental tool of intelligence agencies—so important, in fact, that the National Security Agency (NSA), the primary US agency collecting SIGINT, is believed to have the largest budget of any element of the US intelligence community. SIGINT includes various kinds and a wide variety of information (signals) transmitted by or to a potential adversary or other subject of collection. Signals can come in many forms, including radar scans and other electronic emissions (known as electronic intelligence, or ELINT), or as data or other information transmitted by weapons systems or other equipment (known as foreign instrumentation signals intelligence, or FISINT). The most common kind of SIGINT are intercepts of communications intelligence (COMINT), which is the bread and butter of the signals intelligence effort. Signals intelligence is considered especially important because intercepts of an adversary's communications give insight into what he or she is planning to do. As one director of the NSA is quoted to have said: "IMINT [imagery intelligence] tells you what has happened; SIGINT tells you what will happen."[9]

The role of SIGINT in health and medical intelligence might not be as obvious as it is in some other disciplines, but it can be useful—for example, if communications intercepts indicate that leaders in another country are growing concerned about a disease outbreak that has not yet been reported through formal channels. A number of new technological tools are being used to manage the spread of COVID-19, such as the use of cell phone location data to track individuals who may have been exposed or infected. These tools, because they rely on communications data, can be considered a form of SIGINT.[10]

Geospatial intelligence is the collection of information through tools that are able to observe the physical world. During the Cold War, imagery intelligence (IMINT) from satellites was so highly desired by leaders, and so sensitive, that it was often referred to by the euphemism of gathering intelligence by "national technical means." In recent years the development of many new technologies, including the profusion of satellite reconnaissance systems offered by private companies, has dramatically reshaped the domain of geographical imagery intelligence (now referred to as GEOINT). Geospatial intelligence can be an important tool for understanding and responding to disease outbreaks, such as by tracking the movement of people into or out of an infected area or monitoring the building of new hospitals or other medical facilities.[11] The primary US agency involved in this area of intelligence is the National-Geospatial-Intelligence Agency (NGA).[12]

A less-well-known area of intelligence is measurement and signatures intelligence (MASINT). This is a highly technical discipline that focuses on the emissions given off by weapons systems, by human structures such as factories, or by natural and environmental phenomena. Through the patterns of these emissions—the signatures—analysts can identify the activity involved. While no separate MASINT agency exists within the US intelligence system, one prominent expert has described MASINT as "a potentially important INT still struggling for recognition."[13] MASINT has to date not played a significant

role in detection and warning of health threats, although there are promising technologies being studied that in the future could help to detect disease signatures—including COVID-19—from a distance.[14]

Another key source is open-source intelligence (OSINT). Although intelligence agencies have long collected information from open and unclassified sources, OSINT has traditionally been viewed as secondary to—and not quite as respectable as—classified sources. In the area of health intelligence, however, because so much information is publicly available in the media and elsewhere, OSINT can be especially useful in detecting early indications of outbreaks or tracking the spread of infection.[15]

Finally, a new type of intelligence, social media intelligence (SOCMINT), has become increasingly important in recent years with the explosion of information available online and through tools such as Facebook, Instagram, and Twitter. SOCMINT has become particularly important in domestic and homeland security, but it is also useful in the collection of traditional national security intelligence.[16] SOCMINT is very closely related to open-source intelligence, and some might consider it a subset of OSINT. However one defines it, the use of open-source and social media intelligence has exploded in the post-9/11 era, and the threat from diseases and other health problems is an area where these tools can be particularly useful.[17] As shall be seen in chapter 3, social media and social network information has become very important in recent years for disease surveillance.

## THE INTELLIGENCE CYCLE

Although there are many ways to describe the intelligence process, one of the most common is to see it as a cycle.[18] The intelligence cycle begins with policymakers (or other consumers such as military commanders, government officials, or local first responders) who describe what they want to learn; this step is usually described as providing *planning and direction*, but it may be as simple as setting out a requirement or asking a question. The next step is *collection*, wherein intelligence agencies gather the raw information needed to get the information or answer the question. That raw data is next subjected to *processing and exploitation*, following which the data is *analyzed*. Ultimately an intelligence assessment, briefing, or other product is *disseminated* to the consumer who asked the question. Once the consumer receives the intelligence, he or she may ask a follow-up question or set out a new requirement, and the cycle begins again.

This description has been criticized for not representing the way intelligence actually works in practice. Arthur Hulnick, for example, has noted that in the real world policymakers rarely provide the kind of clear guidance and direction that budding intelligence analysts are typically taught to find.[19] And, as Robert Clark has argued, the model of a cycle makes the process appear linear, with each step occurring one after another, when in actuality everything may be happening all at once.[20] In the world of cyber threats, for example, it may be unrealistic to see the intelligence process as proceeding in such a straightforward and methodical fashion, and decision-makers are unlikely to be willing to wait for the process to unfold before they get the answers they need. This view also overlooks additional steps that may be involved, such as when policymakers provide feedback or insert themselves somewhere in the cycle before it is complete. Nonetheless, the concept of the intelligence cycle does appear to be useful as a model for how the intelligence process functions, if only in theory, and it can also be useful for understanding the processes of medical intelligence and disease surveillance.

## INTELLIGENCE WARNING: STRATEGIC VS. TACTICAL

Strategic intelligence tends to look at longer-term, broader issues, while tactical intelligence addresses narrower-focused and typically shorter-term problems.[21] In the context of disease threats, strategic intelligence often assesses the danger from potential future outbreaks and pandemics, while tactical intelligence warns about a specific virus or other disease threat that has already begun developing. A key function of strategic intelligence and warning is to shine a light on threats and challenges that deserve greater focus and to alert decision-makers to potential situations that might require action.[22] If successful, such warning will result in greater resources being devoted to that threat. In other words, part of the goal of strategic intelligence and warning should be to help ensure that collection systems and analytical efforts are in place and ready to provide tactical warning when and if a threat does arise.[23]

## THE US INTELLIGENCE COMMUNITY

The US intelligence community is the most extensive, and almost surely the most expensive, intelligence system ever created. Although few details of the IC budget are publicly revealed, for fiscal year 2021 the total budget requested to support both national and military intelligence was $85 billion.[24] The specific number of people employed in US intelligence is also classified information, but in 2009 the then-director of national intelligence, Dennis Blair, for the first time disclosed an overall number of two hundred thousand employees.[25]

Not surprisingly, perhaps, following a major disaster or intelligence failure the question is often heard: What do the American people get for that huge investment? After December 7, 1941, for example, a joint congressional committee asked, "Why, with some of the finest intelligence available in our history . . . Why was it possible for a Pearl Harbor to occur?"[26] Similar questions were asked again after September 11, 2001. To begin to understand the capabilities and the limitations of US intelligence, we must first understand a little about the scope of its work.

There are currently eighteen separate agencies and organizations that make up the formal US intelligence community. At the top of the organization is the Office of the Director of National Intelligence, which was established in 2005 after the 9/11 attacks in an attempt to bring order and provide top-level supervision to the sprawling IC. It is led by the director of national intelligence, who is charged with the mission of both coordinating the IC and serving as the senior intelligence advisor to the president. Whether the ODNI has accomplished this goal satisfactorily is a frequent source of debate among intelligence experts and insiders. Critics argue that this new office—employing several thousand people who occupy an expensive headquarters in northern Virginia and including such critical organizations as the National Counterterrorism Center—has only created another layer of bureaucracy while taking away some of the best personnel from the other intelligence agencies that do the real work.[27] Supporters, on the other hand, argue that the ODNI has been successful in better integrating the work of the often squabbling intelligence agencies and has led the IC to successes that have included the finding and killing of Osama bin Laden.[28]

The Central Intelligence Agency is the only other element of the US intelligence community beyond the ODNI that does not report to a cabinet department. It was created this way in order to keep it free from agency bias—in particular, to be independent from the Defense Department, the eight-hundred-pound "gorilla" of the intelligence community—and give it a direct line to its number one customer, the president. Critics of intelligence reforms following 9/11 have worried that the establishment of the ODNI risks making the CIA less "central," meaning that its deep bench of global expertise and capabilities might be sidelined. Still, the CIA remains the most well-known US intelligence agency, and it is unusual among IC elements in its broad, global focus, which makes it able to cover all potential areas and threats. It also remains the primary US agency responsible for the particularly sensitive areas of covert action and human intelligence and has had a leading role in US counterterrorism, including actions like the successful search for bin Laden, when the CIA's Counterterrorism Center played a larger role than the ODNI's National Counterterrorism Center.[29]

Three other IC agencies stand out for providing direct support both to national-level policymakers (including the president, the secretary of state, other cabinet departments) and to the US military. Although all members of the IC contribute their assessments to the broader intelligence community, most are primarily responsible to a particular department. The National Security Agency (NSA), National Geospatial-Intelligence Agency, and the National Reconnaissance Office (NRO), on the other hand, exist to serve both national customers as members of the IC, and DoD customers as designated combat support agencies.

As note earlier in this chapter, the NSA is the US's chief signals intelligence agency. Although its personnel and budget totals are classified, it has historically been considered the largest US intelligence agency, reflecting the huge investment needed to create and operate a world-wide network of listening posts and other facilities. In recent years the NSA's director has also been assigned as commander of the US military's Cyber Command, a dual-hat arrangement that helps to integrate the two cyber-focused organizations, but has concerned some about a possible excessive concentration of power.

The National Geospatial-Intelligence Agency, which manages the US government's imagery intelligence efforts, was formerly known as the National Imagery and Mapping Agency, which was formed by combining the Defense Mapping Agency and the National Photographic Interpretation Center (NPIC). The NGA's responsibilities have grown in recent years, as the importance of geospatial information has grown much beyond the traditional need for maps and imagery. The NGA is unusual among IC members in that it provides a considerable amount of unclassified material to support disaster relief agencies, humanitarian nongovernmental organizations, and other nontraditional intelligence consumers. After Hurricane Katrina hit New Orleans in 2005, for example, NGA imagery and analytical capabilities helped emergency responders assess the damage.[30] The NGA also provides map products and other data to help combat wildlife trafficking.[31]

One of the lesser-known IC members is the National Reconnaissance Office (NRO), which is responsible for designing and operating America's fleet of reconnaissance satellites. Until 1992 the use of satellites for intelligence purposes was considered so sensitive that the very existence of the NRO was a closely guarded secret.

A set of five agencies and offices work for the DoD, led by the Defense Intelligence Agency (DIA), the nation's leading military intelligence organization. The DIA is the parent agency for the National Center for Medical Intelligence, which is the primary US intelligence agency focused on health threats. The NCMI provides medical intelligence covering everything from bioterrorist threats to understanding the medical capabilities of countries around the world, to tracking infectious disease threats such as the COVID-19.[32] As one British officer assigned to the NCMI has written, the "NCMI is the only organization in the world with this comprehensive medical intelligence mission."[33]

Each military service also has its own intelligence office, including the Office of Naval Intelligence (ONI), which is the oldest continuously serving US intelligence organization, first established in 1882; the newest member of the IC is the intelligence arm of the US space force. In addition, each US military combatant command has its own large intelligence organization. For example, US Central Command, which manages military operations in the Middle East, opened a new intelligence center in Florida in 2009 that covers 270,000 square feet and has some thirteen hundred employees.[34] The personnel who staff these intelligence centers typically are assigned from within the service intelligence organizations, however, so these offices are not considered IC members in their own right.

The final and largest set of intelligence community members is a group of seven that work for departments other than the DoD. These are the State Department's Bureau of Intelligence and Research (INR), which is a relatively small but highly respected organization; the Federal Bureau of Investigation (FBI); the intelligence support elements of the Treasury and Energy Departments; two elements of the Department of Homeland Security, the Office of Intelligence and Analysis (I&A), the primary intelligence organization within DHS, and coast guard intelligence; and the Drug Enforcement Administration's intelligence arm, which joined the IC in 2006 and was the newest member of the club until space force intelligence joined in January 2021.

## Other Federal-Level Intelligence Organizations

A number of other federal government intelligence organizations and offices exist but are not members of the formal intelligence community. Several of these fall under the Department of Homeland Security, including the intelligence offices of the Transportation Security Administration, the Secret Service, and US Citizenship and Immigration Services. There are occasional discussions about two of these DHS component offices becoming full IC members: the intelligence offices of Immigration and Customs Enforcement and Customs and Border Protection.[35] There also are a number of other important intelligence offices, such as the National Intelligence Council (NIC), which is part of the Office of the Director of National Intelligence. The NIC produces top-level reports (called National Intelligence Estimates, or NIEs) and coordinates government-wide intelligence collection and production, especially concerning long-term strategic analysis. Also under the ODNI are national intelligence officers, who serve as senior analysts for particular regions or topics, and national intelligence managers, who oversee intelligence collection and production about specific countries or topics. The Intelligence Advanced Research Projects Agency (IARPA), which was modeled on the better-known Defense Advanced Research Projects Agency (DARPA), funds intelligence-related research and development projects.

Not separately included as members of the IC are a number of national intelligence centers, most of which were established following the 9/11 attacks in an effort to better coordinate intelligence on certain topics and problems. The best known of these is the National Counterterrorism Center (NCTC), whose director reports directly to the DNI, as do the directors of the National Counterproliferation Center, the National Counterintelligence and Security Center, and the Cyber Threat Intelligence Integration Center (CTIIC). The National Center for Medical Intelligence, which falls under the Defense Intelligence Agency, is not usually considered a true national intelligence center, but that may change with the growing focus on health intelligence.

### State and Local Intelligence Units

Although most of the attention paid to US intelligence focuses on the large, national-level agencies, the post-9/11 era has seen a significant growth in intelligence organizations and activities at the state and local level.[36] The most prominent of these is a network of eighty state and local intelligence fusion centers, including at least one in every state. Former DHS secretary Janet Napolitano called fusion centers "the centerpiece of state, local, [and] federal intelligence-sharing."[37] Another intelligence organization is the El Paso Intelligence Center (EPIC), which was initially established in 1974 under the Drug Enforcement Administration with a counter-drug-trafficking focus but has grown in recent years into an interagency organization that has been cited as an exemplar for other fusion centers.[38]

The decades since the 9/11 attacks have also seen significant growth in the use of intelligence tools and techniques by US law enforcement agencies. The New York City Police Department has the most extensive intelligence organization of any local US law enforcement agency, but many other departments have adopted what is often called "intelligence-led policing" against counterterrorism but also often for addressing crimes other than terrorism.[39]

## INTELLIGENCE SUPPORT FOR HEALTH ISSUES

As noted earlier, the primary US intelligence organization focused on health issues is the National Center for Medical Intelligence, which is a part of the Defense Intelligence Agency. The NCMI is the lead defense agency for medical intelligence, which the DoD defines as "the product of collection, evaluation, and all-source analysis of worldwide health threats and issues, including foreign military capabilities, infectious disease, environmental health risks, developments in biotechnology and biomedical subjects of national and military importance, and support to force protection."[40] Formerly called the Armed Forces Medical Intelligence Center (AFMIC), in the years following 9/11 and the anthrax attacks soon after, the nation's concerns rose about the threat from disease and human-made biological threats. In 2008 the AFMIC was renamed the National Center for Medical Intelligence and given a broader mandate to support consumers outside the DoD, including the White House and foreign partners.[41]

Examples of the intelligence products produced by the NCMI (and the AFMIC before it) include Medical Capabilities Assessments of foreign military and civilian medical systems. The 1988 medical capabilities study of the Soviet Union, for example, was a detailed ninety-page report covering everything from disease threats to the structure of the Soviet health system, to the presence of poisonous scorpions, snakes, and plants.[42] The NCMI also produces examinations of environmental risks that US personnel might face around the world and reports on foreign research and development underway in areas important for national security such as biotechnology.[43] It has prepared assessments of the threat to aid workers from volcanic ash, asbestos, or other substances during disaster relief operations and has assessed the threat from chlorine gas in improvised explosive devices in Iraq and radiation hazards to military personnel resulting from North Korean nuclear testing.[44] Referring to the massive earthquake that struck Haiti in 2010, the NCMI director said, "When the earthquake in Haiti occurred, we put out close to 100 products."[45]

The director of national intelligence is a member of what is called the Public Health Emergency Medical Countermeasures Enterprise (PHEMCE), an interagency body chaired by the Health and Human Services assistant secretary for preparedness and response. The PHEMCE is designed to coordinate US efforts to prepare for and respond to global health emergencies, and legislation passed by Congress in 2019 sought to improve coordination between the intelligence community and other federal agencies involved with planning for medical threats.[46]

The Central Intelligence Agency has long reported on health and medical issues, such as producing foreign medical capabilities studies similar to those produced by the DIA's NCMI.[47] It may be more widely known, however, for its reporting on the medical and psychological health of world leaders. Psychological analysis became well known through the work of Jerrold Post, a leader in the field of political psychology who founded the CIA's Center for the Analysis of Personality and Political Behavior.[48] More recently, much of the psychological analysis is conducted in the CIA's Medical and Psychological Analysis Center (MPAC). Jonathan Clemente, a physician and expert on medical intelligence, writes that the center employs physicians, psychiatrists, psychologists, and other medical experts as well as analysts with more traditional intelligence experience.[49]

In some cases medical intelligence can give US leaders forewarning of coming events, such as in 1964, when analysts were following reports that the Romanian Communist Party leader, Gheorghe Gheorghiu-Dej, suffered from precancerous bladder polyps. When analysts noted that a world-famous foreign urologist had been summoned to Bucharest, they concluded it likely that the leader's condition had worsened, and when he died the next year, as Clemente puts it, "The U.S. already had eight months advance knowledge of a potential change in Romania's leadership."[50]

In other cases the medical intelligence produced is not as insightful as policymakers might wish. This was the case with the Shah of Iran. As Rose McDermott describes, the Shah first became ill in late 1973, was seen by a world famous French hematologist in 1974, and began aggressive chemotherapy in February 1975. Through it all, he and his aides "were able successfully to keep his condition secret until 1979; even his wife was not informed of his illness until 1977."[51] Clemente writes that if US leaders had understood the gravity of the Shah's illness early on they might have been better prepared to handle the onslaught of events that followed after he fled Iran and was admitted into the United States for medical treatment.[52]

Another example of faulty medical intelligence involved Osama bin Laden. Following the 9/11 attacks, analysts searched for clues about the al Qaeda leader's health in the recorded messages he released—and in the absence of such tapes.[53] The use of a fake vaccination campaign in Abbottabad, Pakistan, to attempt to determine whether bin Laden was hiding there was not successful and led to a reduction in people's trust in public health measures (as well as the imprisonment of the Pakistani doctor who ran the program).

The CIA has a long history of reporting on and attempting to forecast diseases and epidemics. Warren F. Carey and Myles Maxfield provide a fascinating look at the early days of this effort, operating under the name Project Impact, in an article published in the CIA's in-house journal that was originally classified secret.[54] The project began when a meningitis outbreak that was detected in China in late 1966, in the middle of the tumultuous Cultural Revolution, looked like it would spread widely. In January 1967 the CIA's Office of Scientific Intelligence (OSI) reported: "It is becoming increasingly evident that Communist China is being confronted with a serious disease control problem. Factors suggest a breakdown of public health measures under the impact of mass movement of people, and perhaps the beginning of a series of new disease problems."[55]

CIA experts predicted the spread of the disease in part by tracking the movement of the paramilitary Red Guards; Cary and Maxfield write: "In almost perfect order, meningitis infected one province after another all the way to the northeast Soviet border, and, as it struck, the movement and activities of Red

Guards were hampered."[56] Intelligence reports on the outbreak were provided to the State Department and helped US policymakers anticipate and understand later appeals from Chinese leaders for greatly increased imports of medicines, and for "barefoot doctors" to provide medical support in rural areas. Project Impact continued after the meningitis epidemic ended, and according to Carey and Maxfield, CIA reporting provided the first warnings in 1968 of a global influenza pandemic that came to be called the Hong Kong flu.[57]

Medical intelligence can rely on many different sources and intelligence specialties. Carey and Maxfield note: "Disease impact predictions require the retrieval and analysis of immense amounts of unclassified and classified data."[58] One important source is human intelligence; Clemente writes: "Human-source intelligence has been particularly important for MPAC analyses. Surreptitiously acquired medical records, X-rays, and laboratory data have provided supplementary details."[59] Signals intelligence can also reveal important information about leaders' health, such as when the NSA intercepted communications between Soviet Politburo members in the 1970s that revealed important information about their health.[60] In other cases analysts may use open-source information such as media reports, or compare photos or videos of world leaders over time to detect potential signs of illness, such as unexplained weight loss or indications of stroke. Occasionally analysts may even rely on the very old-fashioned but not particularly appealing technique of analyzing the feces of a foreign leader. Jack Anderson, for example, reported that during Nikita Khrushchev's visit to the United States in 1959, the CIA analyzed his feces and concluded that the Soviet leader "was in excellent health for a man of his age and rotundity."[61]

Although the focus here is on the threat posed by naturally caused diseases and health conditions, much of the US intelligence community's medical intelligence effort has been directed at human-caused threats such as biological warfare and terrorism.[62] This focus was largely inspired by the anthrax attacks that took place soon after the 9/11 terrorist attacks in 2001, in which letters laced with anthrax spores were sent to members of Congress and the media, killing five and infecting seventeen others. Patrick Walsh has called the anthrax case a watershed moment for the US intelligence community and for allied intelligence agencies in the "Five Eyes" arrangement, as they attempted to understand the threat from biological agents—including the threat from nonstate actors such as terrorist groups or even insiders.[63]

Intelligence warnings about biological threats include one National Intelligence Council assessment in 2004 that warned that in the future, "stopping the progress of offensive BW [biological weapons] programs will become increasingly difficult."[64] And directors of national intelligence have often warned about the biological threat from either terrorists or state-based actors. In January 2019, for example, then-DNI Dan Coats testified that "the threat from biological weapons has become more diverse as they can be employed in a variety of ways and their development is made easier by dual use technologies."[65]

Tracking biological threats has long been a difficult problem for the intelligence community. The CIA's senior nonproliferation analyst testified in 1999 that "biological weapons (BW) pose, arguably, the most daunting challenge for intelligence collectors and analysts."[66] In 2005 the Silberman-Robb WMD Commission warned about the growing possibility that terrorist groups might develop biological weapons, and baldly stated, "In response to this mounting threat, the Intelligence Community's performance has been disappointing."[67] The next year the National Academy of Sciences issued a report calling for more focus within the intelligence community on these threats.[68]

Prominent examples that demonstrate how difficult this challenge is include the IC's failure to understand the Soviet Union's biological weapons program during the Cold War. The IC only learned of the extent of the program after senior Soviet biological weapons officials, including Ken Alibek, defected to the West in the late 1980s and early 1900s.[69] Happily, and perhaps luckily, that intelligence failure did not result in disaster. But a similarly flawed assessment of Iraq's biological weapons capabilities may have contributed to failures in US decision-making in the run-up to the US-led invasion of Iraq in 2003. In October 2002 one National Intelligence Estimate stated with a high degree of confidence that Iraq possessed a large-scale, active BW program, including stockpiles of agents and munitions. This NIE was primarily, but not completely, based on the reporting of a single source, code-named Curveball, who also claimed that Iraq was creating biological agents in mobile facilities designed to avoid surveillance by hostile intelligence services and weapons inspectors. As Gregory Koblentz has written, "Not one of these assessments has been proven correct."[70] More recently Patrick Walsh surveyed the state of intelligence on biological threats among the Five Eyes countries and found a relatively low level of focus across all the countries. Early in the COVID-19 pandemic he argued that this lack of attention on bio threats was likely to continue unless either the pandemic inspired greater focus or led to some other catastrophic attack by a terrorist group, or some other health crisis occurred.[71]

## INTELLIGENCE AGENCIES ELSEWHERE

A number of other countries' intelligence services also include health threats in their portfolios. The United States has long had a formal program to exchange military medical intelligence with several countries. The Quadripartite Medical Intelligence Committee brings together health and medical intelligence analysts from the United States, Australia, Canada, and the United Kingdom, and has been described as the medical equivalent of the Five Eyes intelligence-sharing alliance among those countries plus New Zealand.[72]

The British intelligence community has tracked health and disease threats at least since 9/11, including through what is known as the National Security Risk Assessment process. For years before the COVID-19 pandemic the threat of a pandemic has been high on that list; in 2015, for example, a "major human health crisis" was listed as a tier-one risk, alongside terrorism, international military conflict, and other critical threats.[73] Canada has a small medical intelligence branch within the Canadian Forces Intelligence Command.[74] A report from the Australian Department of Defence in 2004 noted that before personnel were deployed overseas, health threat assessments were prepared by several organizations, including the Strategic Health Intelligence Cell within the Defense Health Service Branch and in coordination with the Australian Defence Intelligence Organisation.[75]

The French military has the Medical Intelligence Unit within its Military Epidemiology and Public Health Department, which follows a medical intelligence process that would look familiar to any student taking a class on basic intelligence gathering. This unit responded to the global H1N1 pandemic in 2009 by collecting, analyzing, and providing information about the outbreak to French policymakers.[76] One final example of efforts by others to use intelligence tools to monitor for disease threats is Singapore, which has developed a whole-of-government model for monitoring emerging events in order to help the government attempt to identify and respond to threats, including disease. This process is called Risk Assessment and Horizon Scanning (RAHS) and is largely a legacy of Singapore's experience with SARS in 2003.[77]

## INTELLIGENCE IN EPIDEMICS
## AND PANDEMICS OF THE PAST

Although all of these various kinds of intelligence reports are important, many of the most critical health intelligence reports are ones that provide warning of potential *future* threats. As the then-NCMI director said in a 2012 interview, "It is our responsibility to tell policymakers and planners . . . what we believe is going to happen."[78] This section reviews how the US intelligence community has responded to previous health and disease threats, including strategic warnings and tactical assessments of specific outbreaks made in the past.

### Long-Term Strategic Warnings

The strategic warning function concerning health threats can be seen in the work of the National Intelligence Council, which has been warning for years of the threat of a global pandemic, most notably in its Global Trends series of reports. In 2004 the same report that warned of offensive biological warfare programs also noted that "some experts believe it is only a matter of time before a new *pandemic* appears, such as the 1918–19 influenza that killed an estimated 20 million worldwide."[79] In 2012 the NIC warned that a novel patho-gen could "result in a global pandemic that directly causes suffering and death in every corner of the world."[80] The 2017 Global Trends report—the last one issued prior to the COVID-19 pandemic—described a future scenario that could include a global pandemic in 2023 that "dramatically reduced global travel in an effort to contain the spread of the disease, contributing to the slow-ing of global trade and decreased productivity."[81]

Other top-level products of the US intelligence community include National Intelligence Estimates and Intelligence Community Assessments. The IC published an NIE in 2000 titled "The Global Infectious Disease Threat and Its Implications for the United States," which warned that infectious diseases would pose an increasing threat to US and global security over the next twenty years.[82] That forecast proved to be tragically accurate when the COVID-19 pandemic developed twenty years after that estimate was published. In 2008 an Intelligence Community Assessment was produced on naturally occurring health threats rather than on bioterrorism and biowarfare. This report, "Stra-tegic Implications of Global Health," argued that "infectious diseases for the foreseeable future . . . will remain the top health-related threat to US national security."[83] Other high-level reports have been published on more specific health issues, including a 1987 Special National Intelligence Estimate assessing the impact of AIDS on sub-Saharan Africa, and another special assessment in 2002 that stated, "The HIV/AIDS pandemic continues to spread around the world at an alarming rate, and the number of people with the disease will grow significantly by the end of the decade."[84]

Directors of national intelligence have also warned about the threat of pandemics in their annual testimony before Congress; in February 2015, for example, then-DNI James Clapper said that "if a highly pathogenic avian influ-enza virus like H7N9 were to become easily transmissible among humans, the outcome could be far more disruptive than the great influenza pandemic of 1918. It could lead to global economic losses, the unseating of governments, and disturbance of geopolitical alliances."[85] In January 2019 DNI Dan Coats warned that a large-scale outbreak "could lead to massive rates of death and disability, severely affect the world economy, strain international resources, and increase calls on the United States for support."[86]

## Tactical Warnings

In addition to providing long-term strategic warnings, US intelligence agen-cies can use tools and capabilities, including human and signals intelligence, to provide tactical warnings and intelligence on disease threats. Such tacti-cal intelligence can help in determining where an outbreak has developed and what responses have been taken by other nations and leaders. This section provides brief case studies of how the IC has reported on and responded to several recent outbreaks: SARS in 2003, H1N1 in 2009, and Ebola in 2014–15.

## SARS in 2003

Although the intelligence community appears to have reported promptly on the outbreak of severe acute respiratory syndrome (SARS) early in 2003, those reports evidently did not receive much traction. Karen Monaghan, then the acting national intelligence officer for economics and global affairs for the National Intelligence Council, has said that at the time she and colleagues produced a series of short briefs on SARS, only to find that many in the intelligence and national security communities were dismissive of the reports. "It's over there, not here," she was told.[87] Nonetheless, she was the lead author of a comprehensive assessment of the SARS pandemic's global impact that was published by the NIC in August 2003. That report states: "As the first infectious disease to emerge as a new cause of human illness in the 21st century, SARS underscores the growing importance of health issues in a globalized world."[88] It notes that "Despite substantial progress in recent decades in building networks to monitor disease, the surveillance systems in most countries remain weak."[89]

The CIA also published a report on SARS in September 2003, calling it the first pandemic of the twenty-first century.[90] The report noted that "SARS has served as a sobering warning about the serious worldwide consequences that can occur at every level—public health, economic, and political—when unanticipated epidemics arise in a highly connected, fast-paced world."[91] While the report observed that disease-surveillance systems had been able to spot the outbreak relatively quickly and praised the WHO's Global Alert and Response Network and the private system ProMED for being instrumental in detecting the outbreak, it cautioned that "the world was fortunate with SARS because the peak of transmissibility occurred after patients were visibly ill; this pattern is uncommon with other infectious diseases" and called for improved disease surveillance around the world.[92] In an eerily prescient statement, it predicted that world tourism was expected to increase dramatically by 2020, increasing the potential for the global spread of infectious diseases.[93]

## H1N1 in 2009

The NCMI has been credited with providing US policymakers early warnings about the outbreak of the H1N1 influenza in 2009. According to Jonathan Clemente, an assessment by the NCMI "predicted the pandemic potential of H1N1 two months prior to the official declaration by the World Health Organization (WHO) and the CDC."[94] The then-director of the NCMI explained the difference between what his organization does, which is warn of possible threats, and what medical experts such as the WHO and the CDC do, which is provide medical and scientific certainty whenever possible. The CDC, he said, "has to be right. We in the intelligence community love to be right, but we also know that in order to provide timely warning, warning in time for the customer to take action to mitigate what we've predicted, we have to be early. And the earlier we predict . . . the less certainty we have."[95]

Publicly available reports from the NCMI on H1N1 do indeed show that its reporting preceded the declaration by the WHO of a pandemic by about two months. One report, based apparently on information available at the end of April 2009 and dated May 1, states: "NCMI assesses with high confidence a new H1N1 influenza virus (referred to by the media as 'swine flu') poses a potential threat to US forces overseas and within the United States."[96] The WHO did not declare the outbreak to be a pandemic until June 11.[97] Other reporting by the NCMI may have provided even earlier warning, but it is not publicly available. According to David Miller, a Royal Navy officer who was assigned to the NCMI, that organization took the lead on intelligence production during the H1N1 outbreak, but Canada, Australia, and the UK also provided intelligence reporting.[98]

It should be noted, however, that by the time the May 1 NCMI report was published, the WHO had already declared H1N1 to be a public health emergency of international concern (a specific designation, discussed in chapter 3).[99] The NCMI was not the only organization to have warned early about H1N1: the outbreak had been reported in early April by several nongovernmental disease-surveillance systems.

## Ebola in 2014–15

The Ebola virus outbreak in West Africa in 2014 was widely seen as a failure in disease surveillance and warning. As one US official said, "We don't have enough warnings and indicators around the world. We're relying on host nations and nongovernment organizations (NGOs) to do that. Most won't report outbreaks because of potential repercussions. There is a low capacity, ad hoc capability out there, at best, worldwide."[100]

Despite some overall problems of surveillance and warning, the US intelligence community provided what appears to have been effective warning and intelligence support throughout the outbreak. Denis Kaufman, a former senior NCMI official, said the NCMI released "a week or so early warning" in early 2014 on the disease that was later identified as Ebola.[101] The warning may have been even more timely than that. Although the outbreak actually began in Guinea in December 2013, it was not until March 2014 that local officials notified the national ministry of health. According to a report from the US Department of Defense's inspector general, NCMI issued its first alert on the Ebola outbreak in Guinea on March 25, 2014.[102] This was only two days after the WHO issued its first report about the virus and well before August of that year, when the WHO declared the outbreak a public health emergency of international concern.

The National Geospatial-Intelligence Agency provided support for the response to the Ebola outbreak. NGA analysts began receiving questions about the outbreak's spread in March 2014 and, according to the NGA official managing the agency's response, "At that point, nobody really had the understanding that this was going to explode the way it has through the region."[103] By July the NGA had set up a working group to coordinate support for the crisis by the DoD and other organizations, and later that year it released to relief agencies and other responders a public mapping tool with detailed information on the geography and infrastructure in Liberia and Guinea.[104]

A number of US intelligence organizations supported the ensuing humanitarian assistance operations conducted in West Africa in response to the outbreak. The US Army's 101st Airborne Division, for example, provided several hundred intelligence personnel to support the DoD effort known as Operation United Assistance. Richard Conkle, who served as the senior intelligence officer for the US military command in charge of Operation United Assistance, writes:

> This mission required an entirely new intelligence apparatus—one that was not focused on enemy locations, preventing enemy attacks, or high-value target tracking. It required an intelligence structure that was able to track and provide clarity to epidemiological trends; was shareable with non-governmental organizations, inter-governmental organizations, and international partners in an unrestricted, unclassified format; and could enable the embedding of intelligence analysts into a system that is historically suspicious of DoD intelligence personnel and operations.[105]

Conkle and his staff arrived in Liberia assuming that they would be focused on traditional military intelligence missions such as providing security for their own forces. They learned that the situation on the ground was stable, but the most important intelligence need was to identify the spread of the disease. They subsequently embedded intelligence personnel within the Liberian Ministry of Health and at the National Ebola Operations Center, where they applied traditional intelligence concepts, such as the development of a common operational picture, to meet the information and intelligence needs of US, Liberian, and international leaders. They worked not only to track the spread of the disease but also to provide emergency responders with basic situational information like the location of medical treatment facilities, community care centers, and possible helicopter landing zones.[106]

## CONCLUSION

Many agencies within the US intelligence community have addressed medical intelligence and health issues in the past. Most often the IC has served a largely strategic role, providing warning of potential threats and helping decision-makers understand the threat of pandemics and other health issues within the broader context of other pressing national security, political, and economic issues.[107] In the cases of H1N1 and Ebola, intelligence agencies have also served a more operational or even tactical function, providing early warning of outbreaks and assisting in response efforts.

Traditional intelligence agencies do not, however, have the primary responsibility for providing intelligence and warning on diseases and other health threats. Even in the era of COVID-19, these agencies and organizations—with a few exceptions, such as the National Center for Medical Intelligence—will continue to focus on the national and international security threats for which they were created. The job of collecting, analyzing, and disseminating intelligence on diseases like COVID-19 belongs mostly to a system that is even larger and more complex than the US intelligence community's: the system of medical and public health intelligence and surveillance.

## NOTES

1. A useful short summary is Michael S. Baker et al., "The Intersection of Global Health, Military Medical Intelligence, and National Security in the Management of Transboundary Hazards and Outbreaks," *Security/Nexus Perspectives*, Asia-Pacific Center for Security Studies, July 1, 2020, https://apcss.org/nexus_articles /the-intersection-of-global-health-military-medical-intelligence-and-national -security-in-the-management-of-transboundary-hazards-and-outbreaks/. See also Michael E. DeVine, "Intelligence Community Support to Pandemic Preparedness and Response," Congressional Research Service, May 6, 2020, https://crsreports .congress.gov/product/pdf/IF/IF11537.
2. Carey and Maxfield, "Intelligence Implications of Disease."
3. Frommelt, "Defense Watch."
4. Lowenthal, *Intelligence*, 384.
5. Lowenthal, 385.
6. David Omand, "Will the Intelligence Agencies Spot the Next Outbreak?," *The Article*, May 18, 2020, https://www.thearticle.com/will-the-intelligence-agencies-spot -the-next-outbreak.
7. Another function that is closely related to human intelligence is *covert action*, which the US government defines as activity designed to influence events and conditions abroad. This is one of the most controversial aspects of intelligence, but it is a different kind of activity than the fundamental business of intelligence gathering examined here: the collection, analysis, and dissemination of information and intelligence to decision-makers.

8. For example, on the application of open HUMINT, see Bernard and Sullivan, "The Use of HUMINT in Epidemics." On the use of HUMINT by the CIA, see, for example, Clemente, "CIA's Medical and Psychological Analysis Center"; and Carey and Maxfield, "Intelligence Implications of Disease."

9. Lowenthal, *Intelligence*, 116.

10. Bernard, Bowsher, and Sullivan, "COVID-19 and the Rise."

11. For useful background, see Saran et al., "Review of Geospatial Technology."

12. For a recent comprehensive examination of geospatial intelligence, see R. Clark, *Geospatial Intelligence*.

13. Lowenthal, *Intelligence*, 125.

14. "DARPA's Plan for an Airborne COVID Detector," *GCN News*, November 6, 2020, https://gcn.com/articles/2020/11/06/darpa-sensars-covid-detection.aspx?m=1.

15. Bernard et al., "Intelligence and Global Health."

16. Omand, Bartlett, and Miller, "Introducing Social Media Intelligence"; Julian E. Barnes, "U.S. Military Plugs Into Social Media for Intelligence Gathering," *Wall Street Journal*, August 6, 2014, https://www.wsj.com/articles/u-s-military-plugs-into-social-media-for-intelligence-gathering-1407346557.

17. See, for example, Bernard et al., "Intelligence and Global Health."

18. Lowenthal, *Intelligence*, 78–80.

19. Hulnick, "What's Wrong."

20. Clark, *Intelligence Analysis*.

21. Dahl, *Intelligence and Surprise Attack*, 22.

22. On what has been called "opportunity warning," see Gentry and Gordon, *Strategic Warning Intelligence*, 211–12.

23. Dahl, *Intelligence and Surprise Attack*, 179.

24. Michael E. DeVine, "Defense Primer: Budgeting for National and Defense Intelligence," Congressional Research Service, December 30, 2020, https://fas.org/sgp/crs/natsec/IF10524.pdf.

25. Siobhan Gorman, "Spy Chief Says U.S. Hunting al Qaeda More Effectively," *Wall Street Journal (Online)*, September 17, 2009, https://www.wsj.com/articles/SB125305510769813787#printMode.

26. Cited in Kahn, "The Intelligence Failure," 148.

27. For an example of a critical view of the ODNI's contributions, see Gentry, "Has the ODNI Improved?"

28. For former DNI James Clapper's view, see Johnson, "A Conversation."

29. Dahl, "Finding Bin Laden."

30. Petitjean, "Intelligence Support."

31. National Geospatial-Intelligence Agency landing page, accessed December 28, 2021, https://nga.maps.arcgis.com/home/index.html.

32. For useful background, see Clemente, "Medical Intelligence"; Michaud, "National Center for Medical Intelligence."

33. D. Miller, "The US Defense Intelligence Agency's," 90.

34. U.S. Central Command Public Affairs, "U.S. Central Command Officially Opens the Joint Intelligence Operations Center," September 2, 2009, https://www.macdill.af.mil/News/Article-Display/Article/232375/us-central-command-officially-opens-the-joint-intelligence-operations-center/.

35. Betsy Swan, "ICE Wants to Be an Intelligence Agency under Trump," *Daily Beast*, February 7, 2018, https://www.thedailybeast.com/ice-wants-to-be-an-intelligence

-agency-under-trump; US House of Representatives Committee on Homeland Security, "Reviewing the Department of Homeland Security's Intelligence Enterprise: Majority Staff Report," December 2016, 13, https://www.hsdl.org/?view&did =797351.

36. Dahl, "The Localization of Intelligence."
37. "Remarks by Homeland Security Secretary Janet Napolitano to the National Fusion Center Conference in Kansas City, MO, on March 11, 2009," https://www.dhs.gov /news/2009/03/13/napolitanos-remarks-national-fusion-center-conference.
38. Van Puyvelde, "Fusing Drug Enforcement."
39. Dahl, "Local Approaches to Counterterrorism."
40. DoD, "National Center for Medical Intelligence (NCMI) Instruction 6420.01," effective September 8, 2020, 1.
41. Clemente, "Medical Intelligence," 75.
42. Armed Forces Intelligence Center, "Medical Capabilities Study: Union of Soviet Socialist Republics," February 1988, https://www.proquest.com/docview/16791 49935/fulltextPDF/898EA3D5A14F45CDPQ/1?accountid=12702&parentSessionId =ccwAy%2F9z3F8cYNEf06yFPV%2FqS2XQj%2FRN%2BofTAdUvXhQ%3D.
43. Michaud, "National Center for Medical Intelligence."
44. Clemente, "Medical Intelligence," 74.
45. Cheryl Pellerin, "Medical Intelligence Center Monitors Health Threats," American Forces Press Service, October 10, 2012, https://www.dni.gov/index.php/news room/news-articles/ic-in-the-news-2012/item/739-medical-intelligence-center -monitors-health-threats.
46. DeVine, "Intelligence Community Support to Pandemic Preparedness and Response," 2.
47. An example is a 1968 CIA study, "North Vietnamese Army/Viet Cong Military Medical Capabilities," available through the CREST reading room at https://www .cia.gov/readingroom/docs/DOC_0005647975.pdf.
48. Post died in November 2020 after contracting COVID-19. See Clay Risen, "Jerrold M. Post, Specialist in Political Psychology, Dies at 86," *New York Times*, December 12, 2020, https://www.nytimes.com/2020/12/12/us/jerrold-m-post -dead.html, and Tsao, "Psychiatrists, Professors, Patriots."
49. Clemente, "CIA's Medical and Psychological Analysis Center."
50. Clemente, 396.
51. McDermott, "The Use and Abuse of Medical Intelligence," 497.
52. Clemente, "In Sickness and In Health," 41. See also Amir A. Afkhami, "Why the U.S. Must Know the Truth About the Health of Iran's Supreme Leader," *Washington Post*, January 13, 2019, https://www.washingtonpost.com/outlook/2019/01/13 /why-us-must-know-truth-about-health-irans-supreme-leader/.
53. Walter Pincus, "Analysts Seek Clues in Public Silence of Bin Laden," *Washington Post*, April 24, 2002, https://www.washingtonpost.com/archive/politics/2002 /04/24/analysts-seek-clues-in-public-silence-of-bin-laden/a9630153-42b3-46e9 -9e9b-ec871ac63bfd/.
54. Carey and Maxfield, "Intelligence Implications of Disease." Thanks to Dr. Jim Wilson for suggesting an examination of Project Impact. See also Lee Ferran, "Project Impact: 'Disease Intelligence' and How the CIA Traced Epidemics Out of Cold War Asia," ABC News, June 20, 2020, https://abcnews.go.com/Politics/project -impact-disease-intelligence-cia-traced-epidemics-cold/story?id=71299224.

55. Carey and Maxfield, "Intelligence Implications of Disease," 72.
56. Carey and Maxfield, 72.
57. Carey and Maxfield, 74.
58. Carey and Maxfield, 78.
59. Clemente, "In Sickness and In Health," 43.
60. Jack Anderson, "CIA Eavesdrops on Kremlin Chiefs," *Washington Post*, September 18, 1971, F7.
61. Anderson, "CIA Eavesdrops." Although "poop-int" can hardly be considered number one among intelligence sources and methods, a number of experts have discussed it over the years. It was reportedly one of many ideas considered in the effort to confirm whether or not Osama bin Laden was actually in the compound at Abbottabad; see Graham Allison, "How It Went Down," *Time*, May 7, 2012. For a skeptical view, see Jeffrey Lewis, "Who Does No. 2 Work For?!," ForeignPolicy.com, February 2, 2016, https://foreignpolicy.com/2016/02/02/who-does-no-2-work-for/.
62. For useful background, see Lankford, Storzieri, and Fitsanakis, "Spies and the Virus," 107.
63. The Five Eyes alliance is an intelligence-sharing partnership involving Australia, Canada, New Zealand, the United Kingdom, and the United States. See Walsh, "Improving 'Five Eyes.'"
64. NIC, "Mapping the Global Future," 36.
65. Dan Coats, "Remarks as Prepared for Delivery," January 29, 2019, https://www.dni.gov/files/documents/Newsroom/Testimonies/2019-01-29-ATA-Opening-Statement_Final.pdf.
66. John A. Lauder, cited in Koblentz, *Living Weapons*, 142.
67. Commission on the Intelligence Capabilities of the United States Regarding Weapons of Mass Destruction, "Report to the President of the United States," March 31, 2005, 504.
68. IMNRC, *Globalization, Biosecurity*.
69. Walsh, *Intelligence, Biosecurity*, 26; Koblentz, *Living Weapons*, 145–69.
70. Koblentz, *Living Weapons*, 177.
71. Walsh, "Improving 'Five Eyes,'" 598.
72. Tom Tidgewell, "National Center for Medical Intelligence Warnings Gathered Dust as Public Health Struggled to Define COVID-19," *Times Now Canada*, January 11, 2021, https://timesnowcanada.com/national-center-for-medical-intelligence-warnings-gathered-dust-as-public-health-struggled-to-define-covid-19/46808/.
73. UK Government Cabinet Office, "National Security Strategy," 87.
74. Cox, "Defence Intelligence and COVID-19"; Murray Brewster, "Canadian Military Intelligence Unit Issued Warning about Wuhan Outbreak Back in January," *CBC News*, April 10, 2020, https://www.cbc.ca/news/politics/coronavirus-pandemic-covid-canadian-military-intelligence-wuhan-1.5528381.
75. Australian Department of Defence, *Health Preparation Arrangements*. See also Miller, "The US Defense Intelligence Agency's National Center for Medical Intelligence."
76. Faure et al., "How Did the Medical Intelligence Unit Handle?."
77. Gentry and Gordon, *Strategic Warning Intelligence*, 63, 151–52.
78. Pellerin, "Medical Intelligence Center Monitors Health Threats."
79. NIC, "Mapping the Global Future," 30 (emphasis in original).

80. NIC, "Global Trends 2030," 13.
81. NIC, "Global Trends: Paradox of Progress," 51.
82. NIC, "The Global Infectious Disease Threat."
83. NIC, "Strategic Implications of Global Health," 12.
84. CIA, "Sub-Saharan Africa"; NIC, "The Next Wave," 7.
85. Clapper, "Worldwide Threat Assessment," 11.
86. Coats, "Worldwide Threat Assessment."
87. Alexander Nazaryan, "Focused on Terrorism, the Intelligence Community Ignored Prior Pandemic Warnings," *Yahoo News*, April 13, 2020, https://www.yahoo.com/lifestyle/focused-on-terrorism-the-intelligence-community-ignored-prior-pandemic-warnings-182639169.html.
88. NIC, "SARS," 1.
89. NIC, 30.
90. CIA, "SARS."
91. CIA, ii.
92. CIA, 11.
93. CIA, 2.
94. Clemente, "Medical Intelligence," 76.
95. Pellerin, "Medical Intelligence Center Monitors Health Threats."
96. National Center for Medical Intelligence, "Worldwide."
97. CDC, "2009 H1N1 Pandemic Timeline," accessed December 28, 2021, https://www.cdc.gov/flu/pandemic-resources/2009-pandemic-timeline.html.
98. D. Miller, "The US Defense Intelligence," 90.
99. "Swine Influenza," statement by WHO director-general Dr. Margaret Chan, April 25, 2009, https://www.who.int/mediacentre/news/statements/2009/h1n1_20090425/en/.
100. US Joint Chiefs of Staff, "Operation United Assistance (OUA) Study: Joint and Coalition Operational Analysis," August 20, 2015, slide prep 1, https://www.jcs.mil/Portals/36/Documents/Doctrine/ebola/OUA_study_summary_aug2015.pdf.
101. Ken Dilanian, "Coronavirus May Force the U.S. Intelligence Community to Rethink How It Does Its Job," *NBC News*, June 6, 2020, https://www.nbcnews.com/politics/national-security/coronavirus-may-force-u-s-intelligence-community-rethink-how-it-n1223811.
102. DoD Inspector General, "Evaluation of DoD's Force Health Protection Measures During Operation United Assistance," September 30, 2015, 3, https://media.defense.gov/2015/Sep/30/2001714174/-1/-1/1/DODIG-2015-183.pdf.
103. Frommelt, "Defense Watch."
104. Adam Mazmanian, "NGA Releases Unclassified Mapping Tool for Ebola Relief," FCW.com, October 23, 2014, https://fcw.com/articles/2014/10/23/nga-mapping-ebola-relief.aspx. On the NGA's support, see also Calder Walton, "US Intelligence, the Coronavirus and the Age of Globalized Challenges," Centre for International Governance Innovation, August 24, 2020, https://www.cigionline.org/articles/us-intelligence-coronavirus-and-age-globalized-challenges.
105. Conkle, "Intelligence Support," 102.
106. Conkle, "Intelligence Support."
107. I am grateful to John Gentry for helping me think through these issues.

# THREE

# The Medical Intelligence, Surveillance, and Warning System

Although traditional intelligence agencies play an important role in warning of health threats such as pandemics, the primary job of detecting and warning of disease outbreaks belongs to a complex network of national and international medical intelligence and public-health-surveillance systems. This chapter examines these systems, including US medical surveillance efforts coordinated by the Centers for Disease Control (CDC) and analogous international programs, many of which fall under the auspices of the World Health Organization (WHO). It also discusses newer tools being used for disease surveillance, such as artificial intelligence systems that scan global media, internet, and social media sites.

The entire world benefits from public health and disease surveillance systems. These systems have been improved in recent decades, often using cutting-edge technology that has helped to reduce the impact of outbreaks around the world. But the threat of infectious disease has been growing, spurred by the growth of air travel and the continuing encroachment of humans into wild areas where animals can infect them with diseases never previously encountered. Well before the COVID-19 pandemic, a number of critics have decried the international disease-surveillance system for failures in diagnoses, delays in early detection of outbreaks, and difficulties in forcing countries to report quickly enough. One prominent expert wrote in 2012 that "public health surveillance capabilities remain limited and fragmented, with uneven global coverage," and another critic wrote more recently that "the capability for global disease surveillance and rapid outbreak warning appears to be stagnating."[1]

This chapter begins by examining the concept of public health surveillance and assessing the importance of surveillance for public health and medicine: Is it reasonable to compare such surveillance to the work performed by more traditional intelligence agencies? Next is a review of how medical and public health communities carry out the task of strategic warning—by conducting long-term threat assessments and warning about threats that may arise in the future. The bulk of medical and public health intelligence efforts are focused on detecting and tracking more immediate outbreaks and threats through the many types of disease-surveillance systems in use and the organizations that manage them in the United States and at the international level. The chapter concludes with a brief assessment of how well these systems and organizations have performed during some recent disease outbreaks and epidemics.

## THE IMPORTANCE OF PUBLIC HEALTH SURVEILLANCE

Surveillance of diseases and other health threats is widely seen as a key function of public health; as former CDC director and surgeon general of the United States David Satcher puts it, "In public health, we can't do anything without surveillance. That's where public health begins."[2] Sara Davies and Jeremy Youde have written that "surveillance is at the core of global strategies to stop any future pandemics in their tracks before they can cause too much illness and death."[3]

One widely accepted definition of public health surveillance describes it this way: "Public health surveillance is the systematic, ongoing collection, management, analysis, and interpretation of data followed by the dissemination of these data to public health programs to stimulate public health action."[4] Although public health surveillance has traditionally focused on infectious diseases, more recently it has been used to track a wide range of health issues, including chronic disease and other health factors, and even monitoring work-related injuries in Major League Baseball.[5]

The language used by public health experts is often similar to language used in the world of traditional intelligence. For example, a study of the effectiveness of disease-surveillance systems in the 2009 H1N1 outbreak noted that "epidemiologists familiar with the emergence of novel pathogens rightly compare the rapidly evolving facts and scientific knowledge to the 'fog of war.'"[6] Timothy Carney and David Weber wrote after the Ebola crisis, "The common thread underlying failures associated with such public health crises is deficiencies in *actionable intelligence* that inform process, policy, and responsiveness."[7] Medical doctor Tara O'Toole, a senior fellow and executive vice president at the US intelligence community's In-Q-Tel venture capital firm, has described how the work done by the public health community is similar to that of traditional intelligence agencies: both communities collect and analyze data; both attempt to use that data to counter threats to security; both attempt to assess future threats; and both need to speak truth to power.[8]

As with traditional intelligence, public health surveillance is distinct from the actions officials take based on that intelligence. As Scott McNabb writes, "Surveillance, per se, does not include the public health action(s) resulting from the interpretation of the data."[9] But although intelligence and surveillance is not the same as action, both kinds of analysts—whether they are working for a traditional intelligence agency or in public health—understand that the ultimate goal of surveillance and intelligence is to enable action on the part of decision-makers. Henry Rolka and Kara Contreary write, "The purpose of public health surveillance is to support sound decision making in order to prevent or control the spread of disease in a population."[10] William Foege, Robert Hogan, and Ladene Newton make a similar argument about disease surveillance, but their comments could apply just as well to traditional national security intelligence: "The reason for collecting, analysing and disseminating information on a disease is to control that disease. Collection and analysis should not be allowed to consume resources if action does not follow. Appropriate action, therefore, becomes the ultimate response goal and the final assessment of the earlier steps of a surveillance system."[11]

## But Is It "Intelligence"?

A number of scholars have examined the intersection between medical intelligence and national security intelligence, including Stephen Marrin and Jonathan Clemente, who write about lessons that can be taken from the medical profession for improving intelligence analysis.[12] Undoubtedly, surveillance is a key tool of public health. But is it appropriate to use the word "intelligence" in the context of medicine or health? Put another way, although medical intelligence and surveillance systems use much of the same language as national security intelligence, are they truly similar? After all, some medical and public health professionals might object to being considered part of an intelligence system or doing what organizations like the Central Intelligence Agency do.

Rose Bernard and Richard Sullivan have examined this question in their study of the use of human intelligence in tracking epidemics. They note that many health professionals and members of nongovernmental organizations have an adverse reaction to their work being labeled human intelligence, thinking that it means engaging in covert surveillance or some kind of "undercover operation."[13] Nevertheless, they argue that human intelligence—the gathering of information from individuals—is a standard practice for many medical and aid professionals and a necessary pursuit if those professionals hope to understand local conditions and perspectives. Even basic disease-surveillance efforts such as contact tracing, they write, can be seen as forms of human intelligence.[14]

There are many important similarities between the worlds of traditional national security intelligence and medicine and public health, and understanding these similarities can help us improve our warning and response in future crises. But medicine and public health should not necessarily become a part of the national security intelligence system, nor should the national security intelligence community take over any of the responsibilities that belong to medical and public health experts. Rather, all of these areas involve a similar process of gathering information and data, assessing the significance of that information, and providing that assessment to decision-makers, whether they are public health officials or local or national political leaders.

Experts involved in disease surveillance face many of the same challenges that traditional intelligence analysts face, including the difficulty of distinguishing important "signals" from the extraneous "noise."[15] They help decision-makers understand their environment—what is sometimes referred to as situational awareness.[16] Analysts working with both kinds of surveillance systems also deal with similar trade-offs, such as whether to set the system to alert as early and as often as possible (which can result in high rates of false positives) or set the alert levels even higher (which reduces the number of false positives but also risks missing key indicators). In both public health and national security intelligence environments, the choice of words matters when analysts present risk assessments to policymakers. For example, when a public health expert reports that an epidemic is possible, what does that mean? Harvey Fineberg explains the challenge this way: "An event is 'possible' when its chance of occurring is 1 per 10 and remains 'possible' when the odds have dropped to 1 per million."[17] Yet surely a decision-maker would consider the threat differently depending on which likelihood holds true, so it falls to the intelligence analyst to make the assessment clear.[18]

A number of authorities illustrate the task of public health surveillance by using a chart or cycle very similar to the classic intelligence cycle that is taught to most beginning intelligence officers (see chapter 2). Gemma Bowsher, Rose Bernard, and Richard Sullivan, for example, believe the traditional intelligence cycle is a useful model for describing how public health practices can be managed during a health crisis.[19] Some studies have described a public-health-surveillance cycle, while others outline a set of core activities that could be mapped onto a cycle.[20] An example is from Scott McNabb and his fellow researchers, who describe six core activities of public health surveillance: detection of disease through health facilities or labs; registration of data into public health records; confirmation of diagnosis; reporting; analysis; and feedback.[21] Other experts have described the core activities of public health surveillance as consisting of planning and system design; data collection, collation, analysis, interpretation, and dissemination; and application to program.[22]

Although there are many possible ways to describe the typical public health intelligence cycle, figure 3.1 presents a relatively simple model to illustrate how similar the process is to the work of traditional intelligence agencies.

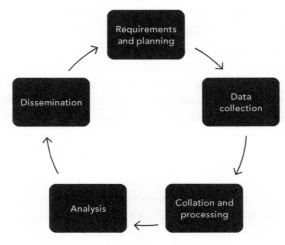

**FIGURE 3.1.** The public health intelligence cycle

## THE DIFFERENCE BETWEEN SURVEILLANCE AND INTELLIGENCE

Because disease surveillance is such a critical part of public health, it is important to note that surveillance is only one part of the larger intelligence process of gathering and analyzing actionable information and then disseminating it to decision-makers. The broad term "intelligence" captures other aspects of the warning and decision-making process that are involved whenever governments and societies face major health threats. The term "medical intelligence," however, is too often used in a narrow sense to describe the role of traditional intelligence agencies in providing information and assessments about foreign medical capabilities and health issues in other countries.[23]

There is a long history of "medical intelligence" being defined as the application of medical knowledge for defense and military support.[24] But we must broaden the sense of the term as it is used by public health leaders to include the functions of the medical and public health–surveillance communities. This more-encompassing definition is similar to the one used by Robert Ostergard, who draws "a distinction between surveillance and a broader information gathering process that involves intelligence and its analysis."[25] A concrete example of this expanded definition is found in Boston, where the Stephen M. Lawlor Medical Intelligence Center was established in 2008 to serve as the coordinating center for public health and healthcare organizations during major emergencies or disasters.[26] The center supported the city's response to the Boston Marathon bombings in 2013.[27]

Dr. Alexander Langmuir, a leading US public health epidemiologist for many years, used the term "epidemiological intelligence" to describe the distinct responsibilities placed on intelligence and operations that would sound very familiar to a military or national security intelligence official today.[28] In one 1965 article Langmuir writes: "There are two terms that are synonymous for surveillance and tend to give the word the broad meaning it has assumed. These are *epidemiological intelligence* and *the general practice of epidemiology*."[29]

Similar terms like "health intelligence" and "health security intelligence" are also often used.[30] For example, Stephen Morse, a professor of clinical epidemiology at Columbia University, has written: "I suggest the term 'health intelligence' to refer broadly to usable information on events of public health significance."[31] The term "intelligence" is also used prominently in the names of at least two important public-health-surveillance systems: the Global Public Health Intelligence Network, a public health warning and information system established in the 1990s by the government of Canada in coordination with the World Health Organization, and the Epidemic Intelligence from Open Sources (EIOS) initiative, which is currently led by the WHO and is designed to coordinate a number of different information systems.[32]

## CRITICAL VIEWS

Although disease-surveillance efforts are widely supported, they do have their critics. Some experts make an argument similar to those heard from critics of national security intelligence: the information collected is open to being misused and can be revealed even when individuals would like to keep it secret. For example, a tension exists between public health officials, who seek to use disease-surveillance information for ethical purposes like contact tracing, and advocates for civil liberties, who worry that revealing personal information— for example, the names of those infected—may result in that information being revealed to law enforcement or made public, stigmatizing those infected.[33] As Jeremy Youde writes, "More surveillance activities mean more opportunities for a person's rights to be violated, for data to be used inappropriately, and for policies that run roughshod over local concerns."[34]

International surveillance efforts are often criticized for benefiting the interests of wealthier nations over their poorer counterparts. Philippe Calain, for example, writes that "there is no escaping from the conclusion that the harvest of outbreak intelligence overseas is essentially geared to benefit wealthy nations."[35] Andrew Lakoff sees the effort to build a global disease-surveillance system as part of a global health security regime serving primarily wealthy countries and national public health systems rather than keeping the focus on humanitarian responses to health issues that afflict mostly poor countries and individuals.[36] Perhaps Sara Davies and Jeremy Youde have expressed it best when they write that public health surveillance is a political act that "may produce action to prevent the spread of disease but it can also stigmatize and publicize those affected in ways that these individuals cannot control."[37]

## STRATEGIC WARNING FOR HEALTH
## AND DISEASE THREATS

A classic mission for traditional intelligence agencies is to provide long-term strategic warning about threats that may arise in the future. Such warnings about health threats have been often heard from the US National Intelligence Council and the director of national intelligence. As might be expected, even stronger strategic warnings about disease and health dangers come from medical experts, public health authorities, and other public sources. Such warnings are often sparked by previous epidemics; after the West African Ebola outbreak of 2014, for example, warnings about future pandemics came from international health experts, prominent journalists, and even Bill Gates, the cofounder of Microsoft.[38]

Some of these strategic warnings come within formal US government strategies and policies, such as the National Health Security Strategy reports and other national strategy documents.[39] Many come from public health professionals, as when the then-director of the CDC, Thomas Frieden, warned in 2015 that "despite progress over the past century, the United States continues to face substantial infectious disease challenges.[40] They also come from a wide number of different organizations, including government advisory committees, congressional committees, and think tanks, among many others.[41] At the international level, warnings about health threats are commonly heard; as two scholars put it, "'Preparing for the next epidemic' has been a recurrent theme in global health in recent years."[42] The World Economic Forum, for example, has frequently warned about the risk of global pandemics, and since 2017 it has sponsored the Coalition for Epidemic Preparedness Innovations to develop vaccines against known and unknown infectious diseases.[43]

Despite this wide variety of warnings, and unlike in the world of traditional intelligence—where strategic warning is a well-established process and is generally sought out by decision-makers—within the medical and public health communities the benefit of strategic warning goes largely unrecognized.[44] Much of the literature on strategic warning for health threats focuses on the role of traditional intelligence agencies rather than on public health and medical intelligence organizations.[45] Much of today's health intelligence effort focuses on surveillance of diseases and outbreaks, or what in an intelligence context might be called tactical warning. These systems are extremely important in the world of public health and they can be put to good use.

## DISEASE SURVEILLANCE

The most basic kind of disease surveillance is used to track the spread of specific, particularly dangerous diseases, through mandatory reporting systems involving hospitals, labs, and other medical and public health organizations.[46] A prominent example is the US National Notifiable Diseases Surveillance System (NNDSS) managed by the CDC. Through this program, data on more than 120 serious diseases is gathered by local health departments and sent to state and territorial departments, and then passed forward to the CDC. Other diseases, such as seasonal influenza, may not be considered notifiable, but can still be reported under separate surveillance systems. In the United States, for example, seasonal influenza is not a nationally notifiable disease unless it involves the death of a child younger than age eighteen or is infection with a novel influenza A virus; nevertheless, seasonal flu can be and is reported and tracked on a voluntary basis through a number of surveillance systems.[47] At the international level, the Global Influenza Surveillance and Response System (GISRS) created by the WHO in 1952 links systems and networks around the world to watch for outbreaks. These traditional surveillance systems do a good job of tracking specific, well-understood diseases. But, as Morse writes, they "are unable to identify emerging infectious diseases, which by definition are unexpected and may be caused by unusual or previously unknown pathogens."[48]

Other types of surveillance, often called "event-based," have been developed to try to detect outbreaks of unusual or unknown diseases as soon as possible. *Syndromic surveillance*, for example, involves the collection of data on potential symptoms before they have been formally diagnosed.[49] Syndromic surveillance efforts increased in the United States after the 9/11 terrorist attacks and the anthrax attacks that occurred soon afterward, out of concern about the threat of a bioterrorist attack.[50]

Disease-surveillance efforts can be *passive*, relying on voluntary submissions from health institutions or others, or *active*, relying on public health agencies to actively seek out data for every case of the disease being studied. A *sentinel surveillance system*, for example, is typically an active effort to test and look for an outbreak in a certain area or among a specific population.[51]

Another commonly used term is *biosurveillance*, which has been defined as the process of systematically collecting and analyzing data in order to detect disease.[52] Michael Wagner and associates describe the term as encompassing similar concepts, like disease surveillance and public health surveillance, but being broader in scope, including the detection of disease in plants and animals as well as in people and involving more than government surveillance.[53] The US National Strategy for Biosurveillance defines biosurveillance as "the process of gathering, integrating, interpreting, and communicating essential information related to all-hazards threats or disease activity affecting human, animal, or plant health to achieve early detection and warning . . . and to enable better decision-making at all levels."[54] *Genomic surveillance* is the use of genetic sequencing to detect the outbreak and spread of new viruses and new strains of previously identified pathogens.[55] Genomic surveillance has been particularly important in detecting new variants of the coronavirus.

Other kinds of surveillance systems are used to identify new diseases around the world. An example was PREDICT, a program run by the US Agency for International Development (USAID) that searched the world for zoonotic diseases—those that jumped from animals to humans. The even larger Global Virome Project, begun after the H5N1 bird flu scare in 2005, has the ambitious goal of identifying all animal virus strains.[56] These kinds of efforts often focus on identifying new viruses because these viruses are known to cause two-thirds of new diseases in humans.[57] Virus hunting tends to be a very hands-on, difficult kind of work, usually taking place in areas of the world where human habitats have encroached into territory previously occupied by wild animals.[58]

Another type of disease surveillance that has gotten a great deal of attention during the pandemic is *contact tracing*, which is the use of a variety of methods to locate and inform the people possibly infected by a person known to be infected. In recent years new contact-tracing tools have been developed that use cell phone locating information to track the movement of individuals, but such systems raise difficult questions about privacy and civil liberties and in some countries (including the United States) they have failed to gain widespread public support.[59]

### Newer Kinds of Disease Surveillance

Because most traditional disease-surveillance methods rely on identification of symptoms or diagnosis by health officials or laboratories, and because they involve reporting and confirmation through official channels, they take too much time to be useful for real-time warning of emerging threats. In order to provide faster and more sensitive reporting, many new web-based digital disease-surveillance systems have been developed, and many of those use algorithms and other tools of big data analysis to process large amounts of information into what might be termed actionable intelligence.[60] These surveillance systems are becoming increasingly popular; one review in 2017 found fifty different systems, and that number has likely increased.[61]

One of the earliest and best known of these systems is ProMED, which began in 1994 as a listserv designed to identify emerging outbreaks. Each report is reviewed by an administrator who vets it before it is disseminated by email to subscribers and posted online.[62] ProMED has been credited with being one of the first to detect the Middle East Respiratory Syndrome (MERS) and other outbreaks, including H5N1 in Hong Kong in 1997 and then again in several countries in 2004.[63] Another prominent surveillance system is HealthMap, an openly available online resource that collects information from a wide variety of sources, including ProMED and news sources. It is used by medical professionals, public health officials, and international travelers, among others, and is fully automated, operating twenty-four hours a day.[64] ProMED and HealthMap have been credited with being the first to alert the world outside China of the COVID-19 outbreak.

Eirini Christaki has provided a useful overview of many of the new types of disease surveillance.[65] Many of these systems are event-based, collecting a wide variety of information on potential disease outbreaks from news, social media, and other internet sources. Such systems include the Global Public Health Intelligence Network (GPHIN), EpiSPIDER, and BioCaster.[66] Another system that has received attention recently is BlueDot, a Canada-based company that uses artificial intelligence to scan sources, including foreign-language news sites and disease networks, to track and warn of disease outbreaks.[67] BlueDot does not use social media posts, but it does have access to global airline ticketing data to help predict where outbreaks may go next.

Other systems use internet search behavior to attempt to detect outbreaks before they can be spotted by official medical systems. Google Flu Trends, for example, began in 2008 as an effort by Google to use search trends to provide what was hoped to be a one-to-two-week head start on official surveillance reports from the CDC. Google Flu Trends ultimately did not live up to the initial hype, and after several studies showed that it consistently overestimated the likelihood of flu outbreaks, the service was discontinued in 2015.[68] Other web-based systems, including those that search social media, have been useful in tracking and predicting the spread of outbreaks, such as with a cholera outbreak in Haiti in 2010 that followed a major earthquake.[69] And crowd-sourcing systems such as Flu Near You allow people to enter their own data and symptoms into an app or website.[70]

Geospatial and remote-sensing tools are being used to track information on the movement of animals known to be vectors for disease or to report on sea temperature and other factors that can help predict disease outbreaks. Of course, maps have long been used to track disease outbreaks, with the most famous being a map of cholera cases in London made by John Snow in 1854.[71] In recent decades the use of geographic information systems, combined with other data from sources such as the Global Positioning System (GPS), has greatly increased the ability of researchers to track outbreaks and even to model and predict future disease occurrences.[72] Other newer systems use computer models and algorithms to attempt to predict the presence or absence of a disease or pathogen in a certain area.[73] Examples include the Global Epidemic and Mobility (GLEaM) model and the PREDICT program mentioned earlier.[74]

Researchers have conducted retrospective studies of these newer surveillance systems—looking back at past outbreaks and pandemics—and have shown that in theory they are able to provide earlier detection than can be provided by traditional surveillance tools. For example, Sen Pei and fellow researchers developed an infectious disease forecasting model built around sentinel surveillance data that includes rural areas and other communities that are not part of a typical surveillance network. They tested their model by using historical data to forecast the spread of past influenza outbreaks.[75] Translating the information from these systems into effective early warning and the stopping of outbreaks has proved difficult, largely because public health officials and other leaders tend to wait for official confirmation of information before they take action. As Avi Magid, Anat Gesser-Edelsburg, and Manfred Green write, "despite their theoretical advantage over traditional surveillance, there is no evidence in the literature that information collection through digital systems had affected public health policy makers."[76] At least one study has shown that, compared to digital-only systems, a system that includes human analysis is more effective in turning the raw data produced by automated systems into intelligence that can be used by decision-makers.[77] (An assessment of the past performance of some of these systems appears later in this chapter.)

## THE US MEDICAL SURVEILLANCE SYSTEM

The current US disease-surveillance system has been described as a patchwork, and one study found more than three hundred separate biosurveillance mechanisms at the federal, state, and local government levels.[78] A study in 2010 that focused on US programs aimed at international disease surveillance found such efforts were managed by a number of different federal agencies, including ones that might be expected to be involved in disease surveillance, such as the Department of Health and Human Services, the Department of State, and the Department of Defense. That same study also found activities related to disease surveillance in places as unlikely as NASA and the US Postal Service.[79]

The CDC alone manages some one hundred different health-surveillance systems.[80] Though its capabilities are limited by the US system of federalism, the CDC is the lead federal government health security agency and the primary authority and responsibility for collecting public health data is held by the states.[81]

The CDC collects data on particularly important diseases such as anthrax, cholera, and Ebola through the National Notifiable Diseases Surveillance System (NNDSS). It gathers syndromic information—on potentially dangerous health symptoms before they have been diagnosed by medical experts and confirmed by laboratory analysis—through the National Syndromic Surveillance Program (NSSP). The NSSP (originally called the BioSense Program) was begun in 2003 to create a national public-health-surveillance system focused on potential bioterrorism-related diseases. Its mandate has since been broadened to include other kinds of disease hazards and outbreaks.[82] Other CDC surveillance systems include PulseNet, which tracks foodborne diseases, and systems designed to monitor outbreaks of specific diseases such as the National Malaria Surveillance System.[83]

Warning and notification systems used by the CDC include the Health Alert Network (HAN), which is used to transmit urgent public health information to federal, state, and local officials, hospitals, and medical providers; and the Epidemic Information Exchange (Epi-X), which is a forum where public health officials can share and discuss information about ongoing health events, including cases of possible outbreaks before they are confirmed in the laboratory. Epi-X postings are checked by the CDC and then, once verified as legitimate, are transmitted to public health and hospitals.

The CDC also runs what is called the Epidemic Intelligence Service. This is not actually an intelligence service in the traditional sense, but is instead a postgraduate fellowship program to train experts in applied epidemiology—or "disease detectives," as the CDC calls it.[84] Alexander Langmuir was a founder of the Epidemic Intelligence Service, although the name was originally chosen by another official.[85] Langmuir himself does not seem to have been satisfied with the name, and he later wrote that "it is poorly descriptive of the broadened functions and responsibilities of the present-day organization."[86]

The CDC developed the Early Aberration Reporting System (EARS) to be used by local health departments to monitor emergency room and other data for disease surveillance associated with large events.[87] It was used following Hurricane Katrina to watch for communicable diseases, and has been used for syndromic surveillance at major sporting events such as the Super Bowl and the Democratic National Convention in 2000.[88]

Several sections and programs of the CDC have key roles in surveillance and intelligence, including the Global Disease Detection Operations Center, which was established after 9/11 and operates 24/7 to detect and monitor disease outbreaks and other public health events around the world.[89] The Global Disease Detection (GDD) program focuses its efforts on helping countries prepare for infectious disease outbreaks and other health threats, through a network of GDD regional centers around the world.[90] The CDC's Office of

Advanced Molecular Detection uses genomic surveillance to track diseases such as influenza and AIDS.[91]

The CDC is part of the US Department of Health and Human Services (HHS), which is the lead federal agency for public health in the United States and is responsible for coordinating across the federal government for medical responses to disease outbreaks. The HHS Office of National Security (ONS) is headed by an assistant deputy secretary for national security, who serves as the HHS senior intelligence officer.[92] The HHS assistant secretary for preparedness and response chairs the Public Health Emergency Medical Countermeasures Enterprise (PHEMCE), which includes the director of national intelligence, and is intended to coordinate federal preparedness for threats from emerging infectious diseases and chemical, biological, radiological, and nuclear threats.[93]

The Department of Homeland Security (DHS) manages several important programs and offices focused on surveillance and assessment of biological threats (e.g., bioterrorism). One of these is BioWatch, a surveillance system established after the 9/11 attacks designed to detect pathogens that are deliberately disseminated into the air. The system involves environmental sensors that automatically sample the air in some thirty major US cities and at major spectator events.[94] However, BioWatch has been criticized for its cost-effectiveness, for producing a high rate of false alarms, and for its lack of nationwide coverage.[95]

Another DHS effort is the National Biosurveillance Integration Center (NBIC). The NBIC was established following the Implementing Recommendations of the 9/11 Commission Act of 2007; it is responsible for coordinating biosurveillance efforts across the federal government through a consortium of agencies known as the National Biosurveillance Integration System (NBIS). As the US Government Accountability Office described it in a 2015 report, the ultimate goal for the NBIC is to help develop "the ability to detect biological events of national significance with the aim of providing early warning and better information to guide public health and other types of emergency response."[96] Regrettably, the GAO found that the NBIC faced challenges in collecting data on biological events and "creating meaningful new information" from that data, and it also suffered from a lack of participation by federal agencies already involved in the NBIS.

The NBIC produces reports that would look familiar to an analyst from a national security intelligence agency, including the Daily Biosurveillance Review and special event reports that are prepared prior to large events such as the Super Bowl and the Little League World Series.[97] It also works with other government agencies to develop new surveillance capabilities, such as the Biosurveillance Ecosystem (BSVE), a program managed by NBIC and the DoD's Defense Threat Reduction Agency, and which collects and analyzes data from numerous sources, including open-source surveillance systems.[98] But a GAO official testified in 2016 that "a persistent challenge NBIC faces is skepticism on the part of some of the NBIS partners regarding the value of the federal biosurveillance mission as well as NBIC's role in that mission."[99] The Department of Homeland Security responded to the critiques by publishing a Strategy for Integrated Biosurveillance in 2019, which established goals and objectives for improved biosurveillance early warning, for reducing the risk of biological catastrophes, and making biosurveillance efforts more efficient and effective.[100]

Also under DHS is the National Biodefense Analysis and Countermeasures Center (NBACC) at Fort Detrick, Maryland.[101] The NBACC was established after the anthrax attacks of 2001 to help the federal government prepare for biological threats. It includes the National Bioforensic Analysis Center (NBFAC), which provides technical forensic analysis of materials recovered after a biological attack.[102]

## US Military Health Surveillance System

The US military has its own complex set of disease-surveillance systems separate from the more traditional intelligence function performed by the National Center for Medical Intelligence (see chapter 2). A study by the RAND think tank identified about thirty military biosurveillance systems and organizations in the Department of Defense.[103] Most of the military's disease-surveillance systems are managed by the Armed Forces Health Surveillance Division within the Defense Health Agency.[104] In 2008 the DoD centralized its disease-surveillance efforts by creating the Armed Forces Health Surveillance Center (AFHSC). A 2015 reorganization renamed the AFHSC the Armed Forces Health Surveillance Branch and brought it under the Defense Health Agency. More recently the branch has been referred to as a division.[105]

The Armed Forces Health Surveillance Division manages a number of programs, including the Defense Medical Surveillance System (DMSS), a centralized system for tracking health care for military personnel.[106] It also publishes the *Medical Surveillance Monthly Report*, a peer-reviewed medical and public health journal focused on issues related to the health of military and other Department of Defense personnel.

The DoD's Global Emerging Infections Surveillance and Response System (GEIS) is a worldwide effort to watch for emerging infectious diseases that could affect the US military.[107] GEIS was formed during the Clinton administration as a response to Presidential Decision Directive 7, which stated that "the mission of DoD will be expanded to include support of global surveillance, training, research and response to emerging infectious disease threats."[108] An early outgrowth from GEIS was a syndromic surveillance system called the Electronic Surveillance System for the Early Notification of Community-Based Epidemics (ESSENCE), which started as a prototype to monitor data from the Washington, DC, area in the late 1990s.[109] After the 9/11 attacks the Department of Defense developed a plan to expand ESSENCE into four major US cities, but the program was part of the controversial Total Information Awareness program, which was closed amid concerns about civil liberties, and ESSENCE was limited to surveilling military populations only.[110]

An example of the US military's global disease-surveillance efforts is the Navy Medical Research Unit 3 (NAMRU-3) based in Cairo, Egypt. It was established in 1946 and has conducted public health training programs to increase disease-surveillance capabilities and improve health infrastructure more generally throughout the Middle East. The unit works closely with the Egyptian Ministry of Health and employs mostly Egyptian staff. During the H1N1 pandemic, NAMRU-3 worked with the WHO and CDC to train laboratory staff from the region to identify new influenza strains.[111]

### US State and Local Disease Surveillance

Public health authority in the United States is largely held at the state and local levels, where there are more than three thousand health departments.[112] The bulk of the basic information needed for disease surveillance is gathered at the local level and then aggregated at the state level.[113] Local authorities also frequently manage high-profile disease-surveillance efforts. For example, the Washington, DC, Department of Health coordinated disease-surveillance efforts for the 2017 presidential inauguration of Donald Trump, and in 2000 the Los Angeles County Department of Health Services coordinated with the CDC to develop a disease-surveillance project for the Democratic National Convention, which was held in Los Angeles that year.[114]

This wide distribution of disease-surveillance capabilities among thousands of local public health units is dramatically different from the way traditional national security intelligence is organized in the United States. State and local intelligence efforts have grown significantly since the 9/11 attacks, but US national security intelligence is still highly centralized at the federal level. The system of collecting medical and public health intelligence is analogous to the Office of the Director of National Intelligence farming out intelligence collection to hundreds and thousands of independent local entities throughout the United States and around the world.[115] Yet, because medicine and public health is so decentralized in the United States, this federalized model is appropriate for disease surveillance and generally works very well.

But decentralized intelligence collection has one significant drawback: local disease-surveillance capabilities are not well coordinated nationally. In 2011, for example, the Government Accountability Office found that although "state and local capabilities are at the heart of the biosurveillance enterprise," surveillance capabilities are not well integrated across federal, state, and local levels of government.[116] An example of this problem can be seen in the story of the BioSense program, which was designed following the 9/11 attacks to collect healthcare data from hospital emergency rooms, testing labs, pharmacies, and other sources in order to detect a bioterror attack.[117] The CDC also developed a BioIntelligence Center (which no longer appears to exist) to analyze data from the BioSense program, and through that center provided support to state and local authorities, such as for major events like the 2007 California wildfires.[118] That program was initially not very successful, as many states and local agencies did not find the information useful, and several experts called on Congress to stop funding the program.[119] Eventually (as noted earlier), the BioSense program evolved into what is today known as the National Syndromic Surveillance Program.

## INTERNATIONAL HEALTH AND DISEASE SURVEILLANCE

As complex and disjointed as the US health-surveillance-system is, at the international level the World Health Organization sits atop an even more diverse network of health- and disease-surveillance programs.[120] These efforts range from large-scale efforts to identify outbreaks in developing countries to focused programs designed to detect and track disease outbreaks in emergencies such as conflicts or natural disasters. The WHO provides guidance, sets global health norms, and coordinates the international response to disease outbreaks. It also has the important responsibility of declaring a Public Health Emergency of International Concern (PHEIC), an alarm or warning to the world community about an extraordinary public health risk that requires international action. The WHO does not have its own intelligence organization, and it relies on member states to relay most information on outbreaks and health threats.

The overall framework for global health security is found in the international treaty called the International Health Regulations (IHR). The IHR were most recently revised in 2005, after years of calls for reform in response to what were seen as insufficient global responses to the spread of infectious diseases around the world. A key catalyst for reform was the 2003 outbreak of severe acute respiratory syndrome (SARS) in China, which was slow to notify the WHO about the outbreak and delayed allowing WHO epidemiologists into the affected areas.[121] This was widely seen as a failure for disease surveillance; as two experts put it, "national surveillance mechanisms failed to identify and respond to the emerging outbreak of SARS early enough to prevent its toll of sickness, death, and international spread."[122]

The 2005 changes to the IHR were intended to increase transparency and improve the speed of global response to disease outbreaks and other public health threats. Member states were obliged under the treaty to develop capacities to detect, report, and respond to public health emergencies, and the IHR spelled out specific surveillance and response capacities that states should achieve. Because it was recognized that many states would not be able to achieve these capacities on their own, the WHO—and its governing body, the World Health Assembly (WHA)—established mechanisms to provide support to countries that needed it and extended the deadline by which states were to meet the requirements, ultimately giving sixty priority countries until June 2019 to do so. Although member states are required to promptly notify the WHO of events that may constitute a public health emergency of international concern, there is no enforcement mechanism—leaving the reporting ultimately up to the states themselves.

The 2005 revisions also called for a broader disease-surveillance effort, including by nonstate actors.[123] Largely because of the limitations that had been seen with the previous surveillance systems that relied on self-reporting by WHO member states, international medical surveillance programs that gather information from news media, internet sites, and other digital sources have grown significantly in recent years. One of the best known of these efforts is the Global Public Health Intelligence Network (mentioned earlier).[124] The GPHIN was first developed in 1997 by the Canadian government in coordination with the WHO; it has been described as an early adopter of big data tools for the detection of disease outbreaks.[125] The GPHIN software scans world news for potentially significant information, which is then reviewed by human analysts. If a possible risk is identified, an alert may be issued; unlike some other disease-surveillance systems that are designed to provide automatic warnings, GPHIN will issue an alert only if the information is verified by an analyst. Another difference from some other systems is that the GPHIN is not a public entity, and it is available only to subscribers involved with public health.

The GPHIN is part of a larger system that was also begun by the WHO in 1997 called the Global Outbreak Alert and Response Network (GOARN).[126] The GOARN brings together national and international health agencies and offices, labs, academic institutions, and others to collect reports—including from the GPHIN—about suspected disease outbreaks.

Not all international disease-surveillance efforts are coordinated with the WHO. The European Union, for example, has its own system, called the European Union Early Warning and Response System (EWRS);[127] a number of other regional disease-surveillance systems are linked through an organization called Connecting Organizations for Regional Disease Surveillance, or CORDS.[128] Nevertheless, most important surveillance and medical intelligence systems are linked in some way to the WHO. These programs include the EIOS initiative, which is a collaborative effort of the WHO and the European Commission to connect a number of public health-intelligence systems and efforts. EIOS receives data from many different government websites, news outlets, and social media sources, and other systems such as the GPHIN, HealthMap, and ProMED.[129] A more focused system is the Early Warning, Alert and Response System (EWARS), which is designed as a mobile and transportable capability to detect and track disease outbreaks in emergencies such as conflicts or natural disasters. The system can provide local health workers with "EWARS in a box," including everything needed to set up a surveillance system, such as mobile phones, laptops, and a solar generator.[130] The value of the EWARS system was demonstrated in Fiji after a major cyclone struck in 2016.[131]

The WHO has also helped to establish disease-surveillance systems in a number of other countries, including in Pakistan, where a Disease Early Warning System (DEWS) was used after an earthquake in 2005, and Vanuatu, where a system was used to watch for outbreaks following Cyclone Pam in 2015.[132] The global disease early warning system includes several far-flung offices, such as the Democratic Republic of Congo (DRC) National Institute of Biomedical Research (INRB), which watches for new disease outbreaks and is supported by a wide range of international donors, including the United States and the WHO. As one report put it, the INRB has doctors and medical researchers who act as reconnaissance units, working throughout the DRC, looking for both already recognized and unknown viruses before they can spread and cause epidemics.[133]

## HOW WELL HAVE THESE PERFORMED IN THE PAST?

Even in cases where disease surveillance has generally been a success, experts have noted that these systems suffered from serious limitations and that the world needs an integrated, worldwide disease-surveillance system to detect and mitigate the effects of a future global crisis. A brief examination of the successes and failures of these surveillance systems concludes by looking slightly further back in time to the cautionary tale of what became known as the Swine Flu Fiasco in 1976.

### SARS, 2003

In November 2002 the first case of what was later identified as Severe Acute Respiratory Syndrome was detected in Guangdong province in southern China. The outbreak was caused by a novel coronavirus—the same kind that would later cause the COVID-19 pandemic—that was found among fruit bats in China, which had spread from wild animal markets in Guangdong. The outbreak was considered a failure of global disease surveillance, and the failure began in China, which at the time had strict controls on the dissemination of public health information and had no national surveillance and reporting system. Word did not reach the West about the outbreak until February 2003, after cell phone messages about a "flu" outbreak had spread throughout Guangdong and caused panicked buying of antibiotics and other medicines at local pharmacies.[134] China submitted a report to the WHO about "atypical pneumonia," and soon afterward it imposed a domestic news blackout.

The virus was meanwhile spreading through several "super spreader" events, including one doctor who treated a patient in China and then traveled to Hong Kong. He infected twelve people at a hotel, and those individuals then spread the virus to Singapore, Vietnam, Canada, Ireland, and the United States. Eventually the WHO's GOARN began to receive reports—including from the Canadian GPHIN—about outbreaks of a new infectious disease.[135] By late March 2003 a WHO team had traveled to China and identified the outbreak as being caused by SARS. Even then Chinese authorities tried to withhold information; Jeremy Youde writes: "During a fact-finding mission by the WHO during the outbreak, one hospital in Beijing loaded thirty-one patients with SARS into ambulances and drove them around the city to hide them from WHO officials."[136]

Early reports noted by the GPHIN had come from Chinese newspapers, and the first English-language report about the outbreak came in a financial news item about a pharmaceutical company that had reported increased sales of its antiviral drugs.[137] At that point Chinese authorities began to take action, including firing China's health minister and Beijing's mayor and building a new hospital for SARS patients in Beijing within twenty days. The outbreak was brought under control within four months of the WHO issuing a global alert in March, but not before it had infected over 8,000 people in more than thirty countries and killed 774.[138]

A US Intelligence Community Assessment described SARS as "the first infectious disease to emerge as a new cause of human illness in the 21st century," and stated that even though it infected and killed fewer people around the world than many other infectious diseases, it caused a disproportionately large economic and political impact and generated outsize fear "as a mysterious new illness that seemed able to go anywhere and hit anyone."[139] The outbreak led China to significantly improve its disease-control system and expand its public health collaboration with the rest of the world. It created a Contagious Disease National Direct Reporting System, which went into effect in 2004, to avoid a repeat of SARS. In 2008 the China Infectious Disease Automated-alert and Response System (CIDARS) was developed to increase the speed of detection and reporting for notifiable infectious diseases.[140]

The appearance of SARS also added impetus to the need for strengthening public health programs around the world and led to the establishment of new public health agencies in Canada and the United Kingdom and to strengthened disease-surveillance systems such as the GOARN and the establishment of the Global Disease Detection Program at the CDC. It also added urgency to the effort to revise the International Health Regulations, leading to the completion of IHR 2005.[141]

Overall, the SARS pandemic was seen as something of a success for the WHO, despite its limited ability to investigate and respond to such outbreaks; the US intelligence community assessment, for example, described the WHO as "playing well with a weak hand."[142] SARS also demonstrated the ability of newer disease-surveillance systems such as GPHIN and ProMED to track the spread of outbreaks. But despite some successes, existing surveillance systems were not sensitive enough and were unable to detect early signs of the threat quickly enough to prevent it from becoming a pandemic. Several retrospective studies showed reports of unusual disease in China from November 2002 to January 2003, but systems such as GOARN were unable to collect and analyze that data in time.[143] As David Heymann and Guenael Rodier write, "National surveillance mechanisms failed to identify and respond to the emerging outbreak of SARS early enough to prevent its toll of sickness, death, and international spread."[144]

## H1N1, 2009

The next major test for international disease-surveillance systems came in early 2009, when a number of cases of flu-like illness were reported in different areas of Mexico. HealthMap was the first disease-surveillance system outside of Mexico to report on the outbreak on April 1, when it noted that local media in Mexico were reporting about a mysterious flu-like illness.[145] On April 6 a private disease-surveillance firm called Veratect issued an alert about an outbreak of acute respiratory infection. This alert went to a number of public health departments that subscribed to the company's service, as well as to the CDC and the WHO.[146]

The virus spread to the United States in late March and April, when the first cases of what was eventually identified as H1N1 were detected in Southern California in two children who had contracted the flu.[147] By chance, the Naval Health Research Center (NHRC) in San Diego was conducting a test of a new diagnostic device, and respiratory samples from the two children were sent to the center for analysis.[148] The NHRC was unable to identify the specific subtype of the sample and sent it for further analysis to a clinic in Wisconsin. The sample was eventually forwarded to the CDC, which identified it as H1N1, issued an alert, and notified the WHO. Additional cases spread to New York City after a group of high school students traveled to Mexico during spring break and returned home April 19. On April 23 their school nurse notified the New York

City Department of Health and Mental Hygiene that one hundred students had been sent home with flu-like symptoms.[149]

The disease raised particular concern in the United States because this was the same strain of influenza that had caused the 1918 global pandemic. The WHO took swift action, declaring H1N1 to be a Public Health Emergency of International Concern on April 25, 2009, only forty-one days after the first case had been detected.[150] By late 2009 the pandemic had begun to recede, and the WHO declared it had ended in August 2010. In the end H1N1 turned out to be not as serious as first feared, and it is believed to have killed no more people than the flu would have killed during a typical nonpandemic year.[151] But the WHO was accused of overreacting and exaggerating the danger.[152] Youde writes that "while they WHO took rapid action, that very speed became a basis for criticizing the organization" for acting too swiftly.[153]

The outbreak was considered to be generally a success for disease-surveillance systems such as the WHO's Global Influenza Surveillance Network, which, according to Harvey Fineberg, who chaired an international committee that reviewed the response to the pandemic, "detected, identified, and characterized the virus in a timely manner and monitored the course of the pandemic."[154] More generally, that committee concluded that "the world is ill prepared to respond to a severe influenza pandemic or to any similarly global, sustained and threatening public-health emergency."[155]

Michael Stoto and Ying Zhang write that global surveillance and notification systems helped to "connect the dots" of cases in Mexico, California, and New York.[156] A study led by Zhang noted that H1N1 was generally considered a success for international disease-surveillance systems, but it also demonstrated the challenge faced by these systems because they will often receive reports of potentially dangerous disease outbreaks even though "it is not useful or appropriate for local, national, or international public health agencies to react with alarm on every such occasion."[157] An HHS report on the H1N1 pandemic found that although there were many successes for disease surveillance, "the 2009 H1N1 pandemic highlighted the need for continued work to close gaps in the capability of the global surveillance network to detect emerging novel human pathogens."[158]

More broadly, the 2009 pandemic offered a lesson about the capabilities and also the limitations of strategic warning about disease threats. The global health community had been warning about an influenza outbreak for years; as Thomas Abraham writes, "The influenza pandemic of 2009 was an event the world had begun preparing for at least five years before it happened."[159] And yet, he adds, "the pandemic that emerged in 2009 was different in every possible respect from the pandemic that had been predicted by scientists and public health experts."[160] For example, while experts had predicted that the next major pandemic would originate in Asia—causing them to focus disease-surveillance efforts on that region—H1N1 developed in North America.

The H1N1 pandemic also proved to be an opportunity for researchers studying the use of computer algorithms and big data techniques to conduct predictive surveillance. Several researchers used predictive models after the fact to see whether they could have predicted the spread of H1N1 in 2009. Although these tools were not used in real time to predict what would happen, they did demonstrate the utility of such efforts.[161]

A final lesson learned from the H1N1 pandemic was the unanticipated consequences of overreaction to warnings. Health experts generally understood that it was not useful for countries to shut their borders in a pandemic because it would do more harm than good; for example, the economic harm that such travel restrictions produce can serve as a disincentive to countries to report outbreaks when they occur.[162] Nonetheless, a number of countries did restrict flights to and from North America, and China and Singapore quarantined Mexicans and other North Americans.[163]

### Ebola, 2014

In contrast with the H1N1 outbreak in 2009 in which the WHO was criticized for overreacting, the organization was accused of sounding the alarm too late for the outbreak of Ebola when it spread throughout West Africa in 2014.[164] The outbreak began in December 2013 when a child in Guinea died of an unknown disease, but it was not until March 2014 that local officials notified the Guinean Ministry of Health about what by then had become a number of illnesses and deaths. Jeremy Youde writes, "It was not until August 8, 2014—eight months after the outbreak began and more than four months after the WHO made its first announcement—that it declared a PHEIC. By that time, more than one thousand people had died."[165]

A major part of the problem was a lack of disease-surveillance capacity in Guinea. HealthMap noted that news articles were reporting on an unusual fever in Guinea in mid-March 2014, nine days before any information was officially released, although its analysts did not realize the significance of what they were seeing until it was confirmed as Ebola.[166] As a group of global health experts write in *The Lancet*, "The epidemic has shown how we are only as safe as the most fragile states."[167] Robert Ostergard describes the outbreak as a failure on the part of Guinean authorities, for downplaying the significance of the outbreak, and on the part of the US embassy in Guinea, which reported the government's confidence back to the State Department. It was, Ostergard writes, "a health intelligence failure in the reporting of information, the assessment of that information, and in the imagination of what that information could mean in a state with weak institutional, economic, and political capacities."[168]

A number of leading figures have described the failures of warning and intelligence in the Ebola crisis. Bill Gates, for example, writes that one lesson was the failure of existing disease-surveillance systems, especially in the developing world. To address that problem, he argues, "the world needs a global warning and response system for outbreaks," including scalable systems that can be used every day but then expanded to meet the needs of an epidemic or pandemic.[169]

Ron Klain, who coordinated the Obama administration response to the Ebola outbreak, writes that the WHO "sounded the alarm about the outbreak too late, failed to develop a coherent plan to respond to it, and never could mobilize key actors to make the response work."[170] Adam Kamradt-Scott takes a more nuanced view about the WHO's role, arguing that the organization was limited in what it could do, since its member states have opposed giving it a more proactive, interventionist role.[171] Others have been more scathing; Laurie Garrett, for example, writes that "the WHO performed so poorly during the crisis that there is a question of whether the world actually needs it."[172]

The Ebola outbreak was another case that showed the tension between countries that wanted to close their borders as a protective measure versus the wider understanding among health experts that shutting borders is not generally effective in containing disease. Experts argue that closing borders makes the situation more difficult for the countries affected, especially in the developing world, as it can make it more difficult for medical assistance or even basic food and supplies to get in. Dr. Anthony Fauci, for example, cautions against closing borders: "To completely seal off and don't let planes in or out of the West African countries involved, then you could paradoxically make things much worse in the sense that you can't get supplies in, you can't get help in, you can't get the kinds of things in there that we need to contain the epidemic."[173]

### Zika, 2015–16

Zika, a virus first discovered in Africa, was detected in Brazil in 2015, where it was associated with microcephaly, a birth defect that leaves babies with an undersized skull. Brazil was at that time preparing to host the summer Olympic Games in Rio in August and September 2016, and the outbreak created fear among many athletes and others around the world who planned to attend the games.[174]

Some limitations of disease surveillance were identified in the Zika outbreak, such as a lack of interoperability among various surveillance systems in the United States.[175] The CDC was criticized for pressuring public health laboratories to use flawed test kits, even though more reliable tests were available—a problem that was repeated later in the COVID-19 pandemic.[176] Overall, global surveillance systems were described as effective in the Zika outbreak.[177] Steven

Hoffman and Sarah Silverberg argue that the problem was not a failure of surveillance, but a lack of political mobilization. They studied three recent public health emergencies—H1N1, Ebola, and Zika—to examine the delays that
occurred between the identification of the index case, the recognition of an
outbreak, and the WHO's declaration of a PHEIC. They found that in all three
cases, responses were delayed more by poor political mobilization rather than
by a lack of surveillance capacity.[178]

Zika provides an example of the potential for newer disease surveillance
and warning systems. In an article published in January 2016, the company
BlueDot analyzed airline flight patterns to anticipate the spread of the virus
from Brazil to South Florida.[179] Indeed, by the summer of 2016 south Florida had become the epicenter of Zika activity in the United States.[180] Other
researchers used information from the web app Flight Risk Tracker (FLIRT) to
analyze flights departing from airports in areas where Zika outbreaks had been
detected, and they were able to predict which US states and cities were at risk
of seeing cases of the virus.[181]

### Swine Flu, 1976: A Cautionary Tale

One more example from the past deserves attention: the 1976 swine flu disaster,
in which insufficient planning and preparation led to quick decisions that had
unintended but devastating effects. The swine flu episode demonstrates many
failures of public policy and public health, but the key failure was a lack of strategic intelligence and warning about the threat of a flu pandemic, which could
have prompted leaders to think ahead of time about what they might do if a
situation were to arise, such as the one they faced in the early months of 1976.[182]

In January 1976 a soldier at Fort Dix in New Jersey died of a new strain
of flu that was later identified as swine flu. Health officials realized this could
be the beginning of a pandemic, but there was no way to know for sure. As
Andrew Lakoff has described it, scientists had only recently developed the
techniques to produce enough vaccine to make it possible to immunize the
entire population of the United States. This meant that "health officials were
thus faced—for the first time—with the possibility of intervening in advance of
a potential flu pandemic."[183] The CDC director recommended a plan to immunize all 213 million people in the United States in three months, and warned:
"A decision must be made now."[184] President Ford consulted leading experts
in public health, including the developer of the polio vaccine, Jonas Salk, who
supported the idea of mass vaccination, and Ford announced the plan to the
nation on March 24.

Despite concerns raised by public health experts and others, including the
editorial board of the *New York Times*, immunizations began to be distributed
in late summer. By December forty million had been immunized. However, by

that point reports also began to come in that some recipients had died after receiving the vaccination and others had experienced serious side effects; and it also had become clear that the expected epidemic had not occurred. The vaccination program was suspended.

One reason for what was later called the Swine Flu Fiasco was that health officials had not considered and planned for the situation; they were forced to react in an ad hoc manner and had not considered possible problems such as side effects. They had also not considered alternative plans, such as stockpiling vaccines for distribution were the epidemic to in fact develop. What they needed, but did not have, was warning ahead of time—what we can call *strategic warning*—which could have given decision-makers and public health experts time to plan and consider options before they were faced with what appeared to be an imminent crisis. Another function of strategic warning is to encourage the development of tactical, real-time warning systems that can watch for the development of a specific problem. This, too, failed in the case of the swine flu, as there were insufficient tactical-level disease-surveillance systems already in place that could have tracked the spread of the new flu in real time.[185]

## CONCLUSION

The United States and the rest of the world are served by an extremely complex network of disease-surveillance and health intelligence systems. In terms of the numbers of people and organizations involved, it is likely that the global health intelligence system is even larger than the formal national security intelligence system in the United States and elsewhere. These systems are not centralized, and there is no clear hierarchy among them; yet they provide an important benefit to us all, as they track disease outbreaks and help public health leaders—and often political leaders—make important decisions. How, then, in the face of these systems that were designed precisely to help us anticipate and prevent such threats, could the COVID-19 pandemic have happened? How well did these systems—both the health and the national security intelligence systems—perform in the case of the COVID-19 pandemic?

## NOTES

1. Morse, "Public Health Surveillance," 7; Hatfill, "Rapid Validation," 529.
2. CDC, "Public Health Surveillance: Preparing for the Future," n.d., 35, https://www
   .cdc.gov/surveillance/pdfs/Surveillance-Series-Bookleth.pdf.
3. Davies and Youde, *The Politics of Surveillance*, 184. A good overview of public
   health surveillance is Groseclose and Buckeridge, "Public Health Surveillance
   Systems."
4. Thacker, Qualters, and Lee, "Public Health Surveillance," 3.

5. Groseclose and Buckeridge, "Public Health Surveillance Systems," 59.
6. Zhang et al., "Did Advances in Global Surveillance?," 7.
7. Carney and Weber, "Public Health Intelligence," 1740 (emphasis added).
8. Tara O'Toole, comments during an on-the-record but unrecorded webinar sponsored by the Harvard Kennedy School Belfer Center Intelligence Project, "Intelligence Failure?: How Divisions Between Intelligence and Public Health Left Us Vulnerable to a Pandemic," May 27, 2020, https://www.belfercenter.org/event/intelligence-failure-how-divisions-between-intelligence-and-public-health-left-us-vulnerable.
9. McNabb et al., "Conceptual Framework," 3.
10. Rolka and Contreary, "Past Contributions," 22.
11. Foege, Hogan, and Newton, "Surveillance Projects," 30.
12. Marrin and Clemente, "Improving Intelligence Analysis."
13. Bernard and Sullivan, "The Use of HUMINT in Epidemics," 495.
14. Bernard and Sullivan, 495.
15. For example, in 2017 DHS launched "Hidden Signals Challenge," a national competition to develop systems to more quickly identify disease outbreaks and other biothreats. See https://www.hiddensignalschallenge.com/.
16. Wagner, "Methods for Evaluating," 315; Wilson, Scalaro, and Powell, "Influenza Pandemic Warning Signals."
17. Fineberg, "Swine Flu of 1976."
18. The classic study of this challenge from a traditional intelligence perspective is Kent, "Words of Estimative Probability." For a discussion that includes public health issues, see Fischhoff, "Communicating Uncertainty."
19. Bowsher, Bernard, and Sullivan, "A Health Intelligence Framework," 6.
20. Moore, Fisher, and Stevens, "Toward Integrated DoD Biosurveillance," 29.
21. McNabb et al., "Conceptual Framework," 3.
22. Thacker, Qualters, and Lee, "Public Health Surveillance," 7. Other reviews of public health and medical surveillance programs that resemble the intelligence cycle include Hagen et al., "Assessing the Early Aberration Reporting"; Bowsher, Bernard, and Sullivan, "A Health Intelligence Framework"; Hartley et al., "An Overview."
23. For example, Bowsher, Milner, and Sullivan, "Medical Intelligence"; and Bernard et al., "Intelligence and Global Health."
24. See, for example, Jarcho, "Historical Perspectives."
25. Ostergard, "The West Africa Ebola Outbreak," 478.
26. Boston Public Health Commission, "Medical Intelligence Center," accessed December 28, 2021, https://www.bphc.org/whatwedo/emergency-services-preparedness/public-health-preparedness/medical-intelligence-center/Pages/Medical-Intelligence-Center.aspx.
27. Deborah Kotz, "Medical Intelligence Center Is Key in Bombing Response," Boston Globe, May 24, 2013, https://www.bostonglobe.com/lifestyle/health-wellness/2013/05/23/medical-intelligence-center-key-player-marathon-bombing-response-marks-anniversary/bVemZLR8CCvdBbIfKfGUkL/story.html
28. Langmuir, "Communicable Disease Surveillance," 684.
29. Langmuir, "Developing Concepts in Surveillance," 371 (emphasis in original).
30. Ostergard, "The West Africa Ebola Outbreak"; Lentzos, Goodman, and Wilson, "Health Security Intelligence." See also Smith and Walsh, "Improving Health Security."
31. Morse, "Global Infectious Disease Surveillance," 1070.

32. Public Health Agency of Canada, "About GPHIN," accessed December 28, 2021, https://gphin.canada.ca/cepr/aboutgphin-rmispenbref.jsp?language=en_CA; WHO, "Epidemic Intelligence from Open Sources (EIOS)," accessed December 28, 2021, https://www.who.int/eios.
33. A fascinating study of the issues related to privacy, civil liberties, and disease surveillance is Fairchild, Bayer, and Colgrove, *Searching Eyes*.
34. Youde, *Globalization and Health*, 147.
35. Calain, "From the Field Side," 19.
36. Lakoff, "Two Regimes of Global Health."
37. Davies and Youde, *The Politics of Surveillance*, 183.
38. Moon et al., "Will Ebola Change the Game?"; Garrett, "Ebola's Lessons"; Gates, "The Next Epidemic."
39. See, for example, DHS, National Health Security Strategy and Implementation Plan, 2015–2018, https://www.phe.gov/Preparedness/planning/authority/nhss /Documents/nhss-ip.pdf; and White House, "National Strategy for Biosurveillance."
40. Frieden, "The Future of Public Health," 1749.
41. National Biosurveillance Advisory Subcommittee, "Improving the Nation's Ability to Detect and Respond to 21st Century Urgent Health Threats: First Report of the National Biosurveillance Advisory Subcommittee," April 2009, https://stacks.cdc.gov /view/cdc/1200; U.S. House of Representatives, Committee on Government Reform, "Strengthening Disease Surveillance," April 25, 2006; Cecchine and Moore, "Infectious Disease and National Security"; and Harley Feldbaum, "US Global Health and National Security Policy," Center for Strategic and International Studies, April 20, 2009, https://www.csis.org/analysis/us-global-health-and-national-security-policy.
42. David and Le Dévédec, "Preparedness for the Next Epidemic," 363.
43. World Economic Forum, "Managing the Risk and Impact of Future Epidemics: Options for Public-Private Cooperation," June 2015, http://www3.weforum.org /docs/WEF_Managing_Risk_Epidemics_report_2015.pdf.
44. Gentry and Gordon, *Strategic Warning Intelligence*. For an exception that does provide a valuable discussion of strategic as well as tactical health security warning, see Wilson et al., "Health Security Warning Intelligence."
45. For example, Walsh, "Managing Emerging Health Security."
46. A useful survey is Park and Reeves, "Models of Public Health."
47. CDC, "U.S. Influenza Surveillance: Purpose and Methods," accessed December 28, 2021, https://www.cdc.gov/flu/weekly/overview.htm.
48. Morse, "Public Health Surveillance," 8.
49. Useful overviews are Henning, "What Is Syndromic Surveillance?"; and Chretien et al., "Syndromic Surveillance."
50. Reingold, "If Syndromic Surveillance Is the Answer?"
51. Murray and Cohen, "Infectious Disease Surveillance"; Park and Reeves, "Models of Public Health."
52. Wagner et al., *Handbook of Biosurveillance*, 3; Hartley et al., "Landscape of International."
53. Wagner et al., *Handbook of Biosurveillance*, 4.
54. White House, "National Strategy for Biosurveillance," 2.
55. Gardy and Loman, "Towards a Genomics-Informed."
56. Watsa, "Rigorous Wildlife Disease Surveillance," 145. There are many veterinary disease-surveillance systems designed to detect diseases in livestock, wild animals, and others, but these are beyond the scope of this book.

57. "Pandemic-Proofing the Planet," *The Economist*, June 27, 2020, https://www
    .economist.com/science-and-technology/2020/06/25/pandemic-proofing-the
    -planet.
58. Leslie Hook, "The Next Pandemic: Where Is It Coming From and How Do We Stop
    It?," *Financial Times*, October 28, 2020, https://www.ft.com/content/2a80e4a2
    -7fb9-4e2c-9769-bc0d98382a5c.
59. For an overview of these issues, see Miller and Smith, "Ethics, Public Health."
60. Brownstein, Freifeld, and Madoff, "Digital Disease Detection"; Magid, Gesser-
    Edelsburg, and Green, "The Role of Informal Digital Surveillance."
61. O'Shea, "Digital Disease Detection."
62. Morse, "Global Infectious Disease Surveillance." See also Carrion and Madoff,
    "ProMED-Mail."
63. Davies and Youde, *The Politics of Surveillance*, 2.
64. Freifeld et al., "HealthMap"; Heymann and Howard, "Keeping Our World Safe."
65. Christaki, "New Technologies in Predicting."
66. Keller et al., "Use of Unstructured"; Collier et al., "BioCaster."
67. Eric Niiler, "An AI Epidemiologist Sent the First Warnings of the Wuhan Virus,"
    *Wired*, January 25, 2020, https://www.wired.com/story/ai-epidemiologist-wuhan
    -public-health-warnings/.
68. Lazer et al., "The Parable of Google Flu," 1203; David Lazer and Ryan Kennedy,
    "What We Can Learn from the Epic Failure of Google Flu Trends," *Wired*, October 1,
    2015, https://www.wired.com/2015/10/can-learn-epic-failure-google-flu-trends/.
69. Bates, "Tracking Disease."
70. "Flu Near You," accessed December 28, 2021, https://flunearyou.org/#!/.
71. Tulchinsky, "John Snow."
72. Lyseen et al., "A Review and Framework."
73. Chretien, "Predictive Surveillance."
74. Balcan et al., "Modeling the Spatial Spread."
75. Pei et al., "Optimizing Respiratory Virus Surveillance," 222.
76. Magid, Gesser-Edelsburg, and Green, "The Role of Informal Digital Surveil-
    lance," 198.
77. Wilburn et al., "Identifying Potential Emerging Threats."
78. Velsko and Bates, "A Conceptual Architecture"; National Biosurveillance Advisory
    Subcommittee, "Improving the Nation's Ability," 4.
79. Center for Biosecurity of UPMC, "International Disease Surveillance: United
    States Government Goals and Paths Forward," June 2010, https://www.center
    forhealthsecurity.org/our-work/pubs_archive/pubs-pdfs/2010/ADA528990.pdf.
80. CDC, "Public Health Surveillance," 7.
81. A good overview of the US organization for public health surveillance is Velikina,
    Dato, and Wagner, "Governmental Public Health."
82. Gould, Walker, and Yoon, "The Evolution of BioSense."
83. Velikina, Dato, and Wagner, "Governmental Public Health," 77–78.
84. CDC, "Epidemic Intelligence Service," accessed December 28, 2021, https://www
    .cdc.gov/eis/index.html.
85. Lawrence K. Altman, "Alexander Langmuir Dies at 83; Helped State U.S. Disease
    Centers," *New York Times*, November 24, 1993, https://www.nytimes.com/1993
    /11/24/obituaries/alexander-langmuir-dies-at-83-helped-start-us-disease-centers
    .html; Schaffner and LaForce, "Training Field Epidemiologists."

86. Langmuir, "The Epidemic Intelligence Service," 472.

87. Hutwagner et al., "The Bioterrorism Preparedness."

88. Hagen et al., "Assessing the Early Aberration Reporting."

89. CDC, "About GDD Operations Center," accessed December 28, 2021, https://www
.cdc.gov/globalhealth/healthprotection/gddopscenter/what.html.

90. Montgomery et al., "Ten Years," 510.

91. Carl Zimmer and Noah Weiland, "C.D.C. Announces $200 Million 'Down Pay-
ment' to Track Virus Variants," *New York Times*, February 17, 2021, https://www
.nytimes.com/2021/02/17/health/coronavirus-variant-sequencing.html?search
ResultPosition=1.

92. Michael Schmoyer, "Testimony Before the Senate Committee on Finance," June 5,
2019, https://www.finance.senate.gov/imo/media/doc/05JUN2019Schmoyer
SMNT.pdf.

93. DHS, "Public Health Emergency Medical Countermeasures Enterprise," accessed
December 28, 2021, https://www.phe.gov/Preparedness/mcm/phemce/Pages
/default.aspx

94. Enemark, *Biosecurity Dilemmas*, 168.

95. Enemark, 171–73; Tromblay, "Botching Bio-Surveillance"; DHS Office of Inspector General, "Biological Threat Detection and Response Challenges Remain for
BioWatch (Redacted)," March 2, 2021.

96. GAO, "Biosurveillance: Challenges and Options for the National Biosurveillance
Integration Center," September 2015, 1, https://www.gao.gov/assets/680/672732.pdf.

97. GAO, "Biosurveillance," 16.

98. Cheryl Pellerin, "DTRA Scientists Develop Cloud-Based Biosurveillance Ecosystem,"
DoD News, February 29, 2016, https://www.defense.gov/Explore/News/Article
/Article/681832/dtra-scientists-develop-cloud-based-biosurveillance-ecosystem/.

99. Chris Currie, "Biosurveillance: Ongoing Challenges and Future Considerations for
DHS Biosurveillance Efforts," testimony before the Subcommittee on Emergency
Preparedness, Response, and Communications, Committee on Homeland Secu-
rity, House of Representatives (Washington, DC: GPO, 2016), 11.

100. DHS, "Strategy for Integrated Biosurveillance," July 30, 2019, https://www.dhs.gov
/sites/default/files/publications/cwmd_-_strategy_for_integrated_biosurveillance
.pdf.

101. Fitch, "National Biodefense Analysis."

102. Burans et al., "The National Bioforensic."

103. Moore, Fisher, and Stevens, "Toward Integrated DoD Biosurveillance," 27.

104. An overview of these systems is Russell, "Contributions."

105. See Armed Forces Health Surveillance Division, "Annual Report 2019," n.d.,
https://www.health.mil/Reference-Center/Reports/2020/01/01/AFHSB-Annual
-Report-2019.

106. For useful background, see Bonventre, Peake, and Morehouse, "From Conflict to
Pandemics."

107. Russell et al., "The Global Emerging Infection Surveillance."

108. Cited in Russell, "Contributions," 214. For useful background on GEIS, see Fearnley, "Redesigning Syndromic Surveillance"; Institute of Medicine, "Perspectives on
the Department of Defense."

109. Fearnley, "Redesigning Syndromic Surveillance," 71, 75.

110. Fearnley, 76.

111. Bonventre, Peake, and Morehouse, "From Conflict to Pandemics," 10–11.
112. Velikina, Dato, and Wagner, "Governmental Public Health," 69. See also Berman, "The Roles of the State."
113. Toner et al., "Biosurveillance Where It Happens."
114. Garrett-Cherry et al., "Enhanced One Health Surveillance"; Los Angeles County Department of Health Services, "Democratic National Convention Bioterrorism Syndromic Surveillance," Special Studies Report, 2000, http://www.lapublichealth .org/acd/reports/spclrpts/spcrpt00/demonatconvtn00.pdf.
115. I am grateful to William Pilkington for suggesting this analogy.
116. GAO, "Biosurveillance," October 2011, 51.
117. Rolka and Contreary, "Past Contributions," 18–19; Fearnley, "Redesigning Syndromic Surveillance," 76–78.
118. Gould, Walker, and Yoon, "The Evolution of BioSense," 85; Fearnley, "Redesigning Syndromic Surveillance," 78.
119. GAO, "Health Information Technology," November 2008, https://www.gao.gov /products/gao-09-100; testimony of Nicole Lurie and Tara O'Toole before the US Senate Subcommittee on Bioterrorism and Public Health Preparedness, March 28, 2006, https://www.govinfo.gov/content/pkg/CHRG-109shrg26843/html/CHRG -109shrg26843.htm.
120. An overview of the WHO's role in disease surveillance is Wenham, "GPHIN, GOARN, GONE?"
121. Gostin, DeBartolo, and Friedman, "The International Health Regulations."
122. Heymann and Rodier, "Global Surveillance," 174.
123. Wenham, "Digitalizing Disease Surveillance."
124. Mykhalovskiy and Weir, "The Global Public Health Intelligence Network."
125. Dion, AbdelMalik, and Mawudeku, "Big Data."
126. Wenham, "GPHIN, GOARN, GONE?"
127. Guglielmetti et al., "The Early Warning and Response System."
128. Connecting Organizations for Regional Disease Surveillance, "Welcome to CORDS," accessed December 28, 2021, https://www.cordsnetwork.org/.
129. WHO, "Epidemic Intelligence from Open Sources (EIOS)."
130. WHO, "Early Warning, Alert and Response System (EWARS), accessed December 28, 2021, https://www.who.int/emergencies/surveillance/early-warning-alert -and-response-system-ewars/.
131. Sheel et al., "Evaluation of the Early Warning."
132. Rahim et al., "The Impact of the Disease"; Worwor et al., "Syndromic Surveillance in Vanuatu."
133. Sam Kiley, "Scientists, Researchers Hunting for 'Disease X' to Prevent the Next Pandemic," CTV News, December 22, 2020, https://www.ctvnews.ca/world/scientists -researchers-hunting-for-disease-x-to-prevent-the-next-pandemic-1.5241685.
134. Jennifer Bouey, "From SARS to 2019-Coronavirus (NCov): U.S.-China Collaborations on Pandemic Response," Testimony to the House Foreign Affairs Subcommittee on Asia, the Pacific, and Nonproliferation, February 5, 2020, 2.
135. Mykhalovskiy and Weir, "The Global Public Health Intelligence Network."
136. Youde, Globalization and Health, 41.
137. Dion, AbdelMalik, and Mawudeku, "Big Data," 211.
138. Toner and Nuzzo, "Acting on the Lessons of SARS," 169.

139. NIC, "SARS," 1.

140. Yang et al., "A Nationwide Web-Based Automated System." For an overview of the Chinese disease-surveillance system, see Vlieg et al., "Comparing National Infectious Disease."

141. A useful review of the impact the SARS pandemic had on global health efforts is Braden et al., "Progress in Global Surveillance."

142. NIC, "SARS: Down But Still a Threat," 19.

143. Institute of Medicine, *Learning from SARS*, 15–16; Polyak et al., "Emergence."

144. Heymann and Rodier, "Global Surveillance," 174.

145. Zhang et al., "Did Advances in Global Surveillance?."

146. Veratect's role is described in Zhang et al., "Did Advances in Global Surveillance?"; and Wilson, "Signal Recognition."

147. The virus was initially called "swine flu" because the WHO's traditional practice of assigning a name based on where it is first identified could result in negative consequences for the country in question. But calling it swine flu produced negative effects as well. The term H1N1 is more commonly used today.

148. Stoto and Zhang, "Did Advances in Global Surveillance?," 24.

149. Stoto and Zhang, 25.

150. Youde, *Globalization and Health*, 152.

151. Initial estimates indicated more than eighteen thousand people died from the 2009 H1N1 pandemic, but later studies used models to estimate that the actual death toll may have been much higher, and as many as five hundred thousand. CDC, "First Global Estimates of 2009 H1N1 Pandemic Mortality Released by CDC-Led Collaboration," June 25, 2012, https://www.cdc.gov/flu/spotlights/pandemic-global-estimates.htm.

152. For background, see Rushton, *Security and Public Health*; and "The Swine Flu Panic of 2009," *Der Spiegel*, December 3, 2010, https://www.spiegel.de/international/world/reconstruction-of-a-mass-hysteria-the-swine-flu-panic-of-2009-a-682613.html.

153. Youde, *Globalization and Health*, 152.

154. Fineberg, "Pandemic Preparedness and Response," 1337.

155. Fineberg, "Report of the Review Committee," 12.

156. Stoto and Zhang, "Did Advances in Global Surveillance?," 30.

157. Zhang et al., "Did Advances in Global Surveillance?," 7.

158. DHHS, "An HHS Retrospective on the 2009 H1N1 Influenza Pandemic to Advance All Hazards Preparedness," June 15, 2012, v, https://www.phe.gov/Preparedness/mcm/h1n1-retrospective/Documents/h1n1-retrospective.pdf.

159. Abraham, "The Chronicle of a Disease Foretold," 797.

160. Abraham, 798.

161. Chretien, "Predictive Surveillance," 380–81.

162. Rushton, *Security and Public Health*, 43.

163. Nuzzo and Gronvall, "Achieving the Right Balance," 176.

164. Heymann et al., "Global Health Security."

165. Youde, *Globalization and Health*, 156.

166. Lyndsey Gilpin, "How an Algorithm Detected the Ebola Outbreak a Week Early, and What It Could Do Next," *Techrepublic.Com*, August 26, 2014, https://www.techrepublic.com/article/how-an-algorithm-detected-the-ebola-outbreak-a-week-early-and-what-it-could-do-next/.

167. Heymann et al., "Global Health Security," 1885. For an in-depth look at how disease surveillance functions in Sierra Leone during the outbreak, see Ilesanmi et al., "Evaluation of Ebola Virus."
168. Ostergard, "The West Africa Ebola Outbreak," 489. Another good survey of the intelligence problems in this case is Bernard and Sullivan, "The Use of HUMINT in Epidemics."
169. Gates, "The Next Epidemic," 1382.
170. Ronald Klain, "Confronting the Pandemic Threat," *Democracy* 40 (Spring 2016), https://democracyjournal.org/magazine/40/confronting-the-pandemic-threat/.
171. Kamradt-Scott, "WHO's to Blame?," 412.
172. Garrett, "Ebola's Lessons," 102. For a similar critical assessment, see Wibulpolprasert and Chowdhury, "World Health Organization."
173. S. A. Miller, "A Top Health Expert Warns Against Closing Borders to Stop Ebola," *Washington Times*, October 6, 2014, https://www.washingtontimes.com/news/2014/oct/6/a-top-health-expert-warns-against-closing-borders-/.
174. Youde, *Globalization and Health*, 162–67.
175. GAO, "Emerging Infectious Diseases: Actions Needed to Address the Challenges of Responding to Zika Virus Disease Outbreaks," May 2017, 33.
176. David Willman, "Lessons Unlearned: Four Years before the CDC Fumbled Coronavirus Testing, the Agency Made Some of the Same Mistakes with Zika," *Washington Post*, July 4, 2020, https://www.washingtonpost.com/investigations/lessons-unlearned-four-years-before-the-cdc-fumbled-coronavirus-testing-the-agency-made-some-of-the-same-mistakes-with-zika/2020/07/03/c32ca530-a8af-11ea-94d2-d7bc43b26bf9_story.html.
177. Youde, *Globalization and Health*.
178. Hoffman and Silverberg, "Delays in Global Disease."
179. Bogoch et al., "Anticipating the International Spread."
180. Fellner, "Zika in America."
181. Bates, "Tracking Disease," 21; Huff et al., "FLIRT-Ing with Zika."
182. Key sources on this case include Neustadt and Fineberg, *The Swine Flu Affair*; and Lakoff, "From Population to Vital System."
183. Lakoff, "From Population to Vital System," 39.
184. Lakoff, 41.
185. On the limitations of influenza surveillance systems in 1976, see Dehner, "WHO Knows Best?."

# FOUR

## Was the Coronavirus Pandemic an Intelligence Failure?

Since the early days of the COVID-19 outbreak, experts have debated whether the crisis was a failure of intelligence. Some argue the pandemic was the result of mistakes made by US intelligence agencies that failed to warn or by policymakers who failed to heed the warnings they were given.[1] President Trump blamed the US intelligence community for downplaying the threat, while at the same time also claiming that he saw it coming early on.[2]

Although we may not be able to make a full assessment until a national coronavirus commission or other high-level body investigates what happened, enough information is now available to indicate that the disaster was indeed an intelligence failure—a *global* failure, in which the complex worldwide system of collection, analysis, and warning that had been developed for just such an eventuality was unsuccessful in preventing the spread of the disease onto every continent and into every country on earth. If we hope to prevent future disasters we must understand why this particular failure occurred. This chapter examines the performance of the US intelligence community and the US and global public health intelligence system to argue that the COVID-19 global intelligence failure was remarkably similar to past failures of intelligence and warning, such as Pearl Harbor and, in particular, the 9/11 attacks.

The crisis we face today is very different from those previous intelligence failures, of course, most notably in the nature of the enemy. But, despite these differences, in both the case of the 9/11 attacks and the COVID-19 pandemic, the United States was threatened by an adversary that was present in the country for several weeks or even months before it was recognized for the threat it was. In both cases the systems designed to detect just such a threat failed to prevent disaster. Today, as in the past, we have seen a deadly combination of three factors at work: strategic-level warnings that preceded the crisis but were ineffective in preventing it; a lack of specific intelligence on the actual threat as it developed, until it was too late; and an absence of receptivity—the willingness to listen to and act on the basis of the intelligence received—among policymakers who could have done more to head off disaster.[3]

We know beyond doubt that the possibility of a global pandemic was widely predicted. The scientific and intelligence communities had been sounding that alarm for years, which leaders failed to heed. Does this lapse in leadership exonerate intelligence and public health officials? Receptivity to warnings is a two-way street. When intelligence officers believe that a threat is significant, they have a responsibility to present its existence to decision-makers in the most effective manner possible. The history of intelligence success shows that intelligence officers have almost always had to work hard to get their leaders' attention. Throughout the prelude to the pandemic, in this crucial respect, the intelligence community failed. It did not take the necessary steps to ensure that leaders understood the warnings they were being given.

From an intelligence perspective, the most important difference between past disasters such as 9/11 and the COVID-19 pandemic of today may be that today the task of analyzing data and warning of a threat is not shouldered solely, or even primarily, by the agencies of the traditional US intelligence community. In fact, the job of collecting and analyzing intelligence on a pandemic threat belongs mostly to a network of national and international public health surveillance systems.

So far we have examined how the traditional intelligence community and the medical and public health communities conduct intelligence, surveillance, and warning against pandemics and other health threats. We now must look at how well those organizations and communities did their job in the case of the COVID-19 pandemic and, in an effort to help place today's events in context, compare the crisis with intelligence failures of the past—especially the 9/11 terrorist attacks.

Concerning a pandemic, the agencies of the US intelligence community have collection and analysis missions beyond the role of providing early warning. The Department of Homeland Security, for example, reportedly analyzed shifts in Chinese global trade data in May 2020 to conclude that China knew the severity of the virus early on, but misled the rest of the world.[4] The CIA reportedly made similar assessments.[5] Beyond the US intelligence community, intelligence agencies around the world have reportedly been engaged in an intense competition to determine others' vaccine capabilities and even steal research for themselves.[6] Since signs of the COVID-19 pandemic first appeared, the US intelligence community has been searching for clues as to its origins—a search that, at this writing (mid-2022) has so far produced few firm answers. All of these intelligence efforts are undoubtedly important, but we must also focus on the role of providing warning and analysis in the early stages of the crisis.

Many intelligence experts have made the opposite argument of the one made here, instead claiming that the pandemic does *not* represent an intelligence failure. This chapter provides a detailed examination of the strategic level warnings that were available before the crisis, and why these warnings were insufficient to prevent disaster. This is followed by scrutiny of the tactical intelligence and warning that was present as the outbreak began and why that, too, was not enough to stop the spread of the virus or mitigate its effects. The chapter concludes with a review of the third key factor involved in intelligence success and failure—the level of receptivity among decision-makers, including in countries around the world beyond the United States—and suggests alternative scenarios for the future.

## INTELLIGENCE FAILURE, YES OR NO?

A group of intelligence experts believe that, if anything, the US intelligence community deserves credit for doing an excellent job of providing warning of the coming pandemic. Some of these experts argue that the blame rests firmly with President Trump for not having listened to the very clear warnings provided to him. Chris Whipple, for example, writes that if intelligence warnings about the 9/11 attacks could have been considered like red lights flashing, the COVID-19 pandemic, by comparison, was "a case of sirens sounding, horns blaring and a parade down Main Street."[7] Even in the face of these prominent warnings, Whipple argues, "Trump looked the other way."[8]

Other experts, such as Calder Walton, have argued that the pandemic does not appear to have been an intelligence failure because intelligence agencies did warn, but decision-makers failed to act on that warning.[9] Gregory Treverton, former chair of the National Intelligence Council, argues there was enough warning, but it was more a failure of leadership than of warning.[10] James Wirtz writes: "It is clear that COVID-19 cannot be characterized as an intelligence failure, or as a failure of public health officials or the security studies community to understand the general course and consequences of the threat. The possibility of a global pandemic was not only predictable, it was also predicted by the scientific (and intelligence) community."[11]

To some extent the argument about whether the pandemic should be considered an intelligence failure or not depends on where one sets the bar for success. How much warning is enough? Studies conducted after almost any crisis or disaster consistently show that someone was warned at some point, and it is a truism in the intelligence business that after a surprise event, indicators are always found in the pipeline.[12] Even so, few would argue that an intelligence (or public health) agency should be given a pass just because a threat was briefly mentioned in a report or cited in testimony.

Perhaps intelligence "failure" is not so much a matter of whether a warning was given—since, after all, modern intelligence systems tend to warn often about almost everything—but rather a matter of whether intelligence agencies and officials were focused on the right problems and truly doing the best job they could. This was the argument then-director of central intelligence George Tenet made in 2002 when he testified that the 9/11 attacks had not been a case of intelligence failure. As he said, "When people use the word 'failure,' 'failure' means no focus, no attention, no discipline—and those were not present in what either we or the FBI did here and around the world."[13] Tenet's defense of the intelligence community he was leading is understandable, but he set the bar for success too low. It is not enough for intelligence agencies and officials to be focused and disciplined. Their job is to collect, analyze, and convey intelligence and warning to decision-makers in order to anticipate or mitigate threats. When those do not happen, the result is an intelligence failure, even though all personnel involved may have been doing the best they could.

A second argument often made about intelligence failure is that it is often the fault of decision-makers or other customers, who fail to heed the warnings they are given. According to this logic, the job of intelligence officials is to warn, and once that mission is accomplished, the final result is out of their hands. If leaders are not receptive, the error is theirs alone, and any resulting disaster is their fault. This is a commonly held belief among intelligence professionals and experts, and it does make sense. After all, it is indeed the job of senior decision-makers, including elected officials and military commanders, to decide what to do with the intelligence warnings they receive. But this, too, is setting the bar too low. The goal of intelligence should not be simply to warn—it should be to help leaders and policymakers avoid disaster. The final decisions, of course, are made by leaders and not by analysts; but experience has shown that intelligence analysts can and must be ready to push harder if they feel their warnings are not being heard. From what we know so far in the case of the COVID-19 pandemic, few pushed and even fewer were heard.

## WARNINGS BEFORE THE CRISIS

In the cases of both the 9/11 attacks and the COVID-19 outbreak, strategic-level, big-picture warnings were made long before the disasters from prominent officials and blue-ribbon commissions, all of which went unheeded. There were also tabletop exercises and wargames that, after the fact, seem remarkably prescient. How could so many warnings by so many experts have failed to prevent these crises? Experience has shown that this kind of warning actually does very little to prevent a disaster, because decision-makers are unlikely to take expensive, potentially risky actions based on general warning of possible events. This section begins with a review of the many warnings that came in before the COVID-19 outbreak happened, from both traditional national security intelligence sources and from medical and public health experts, then places these warnings in the context of similar warnings in the case of the 9/11 attacks. It then examines why these warnings failed.

## Strategic Warnings

A major disaster such as the COVID-19 pandemic or the 9/11 attacks rarely occurs without warning. Before 9/11, for example, White House counter-terrorism advisor Richard A. Clarke famously warned of the threat from al Qaeda, and as the *9/11 Commission Report* notes, multiple commissions and studies warned about the danger of terrorist attacks well before September 11. Before the pandemic, warnings of the danger from an infectious disease outbreak came from individuals as well known as Bill Gates and from studies such as a blue-ribbon report published in November 2019 by the CSIS Commission on Strengthening America's Health Security, which warned that "the American people are far from safe. To the contrary, the United States remains woefully ill-prepared to respond to global health security threats."[14]

Warnings about the danger of pandemics have been sounded for decades, by journalists such as Laurie Garrett, scholars such as Michael T. Osterholm, and many others.[15] To name just one example of these early warnings, in 2003 a report by the Institute of Medicine warned of the threat from newly discovered infectious diseases and cautioned that existing systems for disease surveillance were insufficient. It called for the United States to lead an effort to develop a global system of disease surveillance.[16]

Some of these warnings focused on the threat of bioterrorism, while many others warned about the danger from naturally occurring infectious disease. Former Barack Obama administration Ebola czar (and current Biden administration chief of staff) Ronald Klain warned in 2016 that the single most likely catastrophe that could confront the incoming Trump administration was a pandemic illness.[17] These warnings grew even more strident as the COVID-19 outbreak neared; in September 2019 the Global Preparedness Monitoring Board, in a report prepared for the World Health Organization, called for greater effort by the international community to prepare for global health crises.[18] In October 2019 the Nuclear Threat Initiative published its Global Health Security Index, warning that "no country is fully prepared for epidemics or pandemics," although the same report ranked the United States as number 1 out of 195 countries in terms of pandemic readiness.[19]

Warnings about threats also come from war games, exercises, and scenarios used by government agencies, think tanks, and scholars to imagine future dangers and attempt to prepare for them. Well before the 9/11 attacks, for example, a number of war games and simulations examined the possibility that terrorists might use airplanes as bombs. The COVID-19 outbreak was just as extensively war-gamed and anticipated; the Department of Health and Human

Services ran an exercise called Crimson Contagion throughout much of 2019 that involved twelve states and a dozen federal agencies.[20] The scenario for that exercise involved a pandemic flu outbreak that began in China and was brought to the United States by a tourist from Chicago.

Many of these scenarios seem to have anticipated what the world went through only a short while later. The Federal Emergency Management Agency (FEMA) published a national threat assessment in July 2019 that described a scenario in which a novel flu virus is discovered in Washington, DC, and within weeks spreads throughout the country and around the world, forcing businesses to close, overwhelming medical facilities, and leading to widespread civil disorder.[21] Later in 2019 incoming Trump administration senior personnel participated with outgoing Obama officials in a tabletop exercise that tested their responses to a global flu pandemic.[22] Then in September 2019 the US Naval War College and Johns Hopkins University hosted a war game called "Urban Outbreak 2019" in which military, public health, and emergency response professionals simulated the decision-making needed to respond to a major infectious disease outbreak in a large global city. They found that local responses and containment efforts would likely break down quickly, requiring a global response.[23]

In October 2019, just months before the COVID-19 outbreak, the Johns Hopkins Center for Health Security, the World Economic Forum, and the Bill & Melinda Gates Foundation war-gamed what would happen if a new disease swept the globe. Their tabletop exercise found that "the next severe pandemic will not only cause great illness and loss of life but could also trigger major cascading economic and societal consequences that could contribute greatly to global impact and suffering."[24]

Strategic warnings also come from the many organizations that make up the US intelligence community. Before 9/11, agencies as well known as the Central Intelligence Agency and as obscure as the intelligence office of the Federal Aviation Administration warned about a rising terrorist threat. Many of those same agencies have been warning for years about health threats. In January 2000 the US intelligence community published a National Intelligence Estimate that warned infectious diseases "will endanger US citizens at home and abroad, threaten US armed forces deployed overseas, and exacerbate social and political instability in key countries and regions in which the United States has significant interests."[25]

The US National Intelligence Council (NIC), the body that coordinates top-level estimates and reports, has been highlighting the pandemic threat for years in its series of Global Trends reports.[26] In 2008, for example, the NIC published Global Trends 2025, which includes a shockingly prescient scenario of how in 2025 a zoonotic pathogen might emerge in an area of high population density and close association between humans and animals, such as in many parts of China and Southeast Asia. The resulting pandemic, the NIC warns, would produce as many as tens of millions of deaths in the United States alone.[27] In 2012 the NIC published Global Trends 2030, which calls a pandemic a "potential black swan" and warns that "an easily transmissible novel respiratory pathogen that kills or incapacitates more than one percent of its victims is among the most disruptive events possible. Such an outbreak could result in millions of people suffering and dying in every corner of the world in less than six months."[28]

Directors of national intelligence have been warning about the threat from pandemics. James Clapper testified before the Senate in 2015 that "if a highly pathogenic avian influenza virus like H7N9 were to become easily transmissible among humans, the outcome could be far more disruptive than the great influenza pandemic of 1918. It could lead to global economic losses, the unseating of governments, and disturbance of geopolitical alliances."[29] Nearly a year before the current outbreak, then-DNI Dan Coats warned in January 2019 that "the United States and the world will remain vulnerable to the next flu pandemic or large-scale outbreak of a contagious disease that could lead to massive rates of death and disability."[30] The DNI's February 2020 annual threat assessment report was not delivered to Congress (amid disagreements between President Trump and the intelligence community), but reportedly the DNI's statement would have contained similar wording about pandemics as found in the previous year's report.[31]

Similar ominous strategic warnings have been heard from health experts at the international level. The WHO, for example, in 2018 published a list of disease threats, including what it called Disease X, which "represents the knowledge that a serious international epidemic could be caused by a pathogen currently unknown to cause human disease."[32]

## Why Were Warnings Missed?

Scholars, journalists, and others have asked the question: How could this disaster have happened, when it was so clearly foreseen? The *Washington Post* put it this way: "The question that must be addressed in future postmortems is why all this expertise and warning was ignored."[33]

Part of the answer lies in human psychology: we are all surprisingly easy to surprise. As Harvard professor Jeffrey Frankel has noted, human beings, including experts, are often taken by surprise when rare or extreme events happen, even when those events have been foreseen.[34] The disregard of strategic warnings in the years before the current pandemic can also be partly explained as one example of the broader disregard of expert and scientific advice within the Trump administration.[35]

As seen in the history of intelligence and surprise, however, such broad, strategic warnings are actually quite ineffective in preventing disaster.[36] In a previous book examining the intelligence failures of Pearl Harbor and 9/11, I show that early warnings often appear after the fact to have been eerily prophetic.[37] But it is not enough for intelligence agencies simply to warn of threats that may come. For one thing, decision-makers—especially at senior levels—get a great many of these warnings. In the same testimony in which the DNI warned of the pandemic threat in early 2019, he also warned of increasing threats: from cyber attacks, from weapons of mass destruction, from environmental change, and from more dangers to come. Even if a senior leader vowed to take seriously every threat brought to her or his attention (a foolhardy endeavor to be sure), how would that leader decide where to start?

The second reason these kinds of big-picture strategic warnings are ineffective in preventing threats from developing is that decision-makers—again, especially senior leaders—tend to be reluctant to devote resources and spend their limited capital on threats that simply *might* appear *someday*. Specific intelligence is needed before they reasonably can be expected to decide how and where to take action when faced with such a panoply of threats. In order to use intelligence to prevent disaster and surprise, leaders need specific, credible threat information—what we call tactical intelligence—before they can respond effectively.

## ALARMS AS A CRISIS DEVELOPS

In the early weeks and months of the COVID-19 crisis, just as in the run-up to the 9/11 attacks, intelligence agencies were warning of the rising threat. In both cases the specific, tactical-level intelligence on an actual threat—the 9/11 hijacking plot and the novel coronavirus—was frustratingly and tragically limited. The tactical warnings from the traditional national security intelligence community and from the medical and public health communities were simply not enough.

### *Tactical Warnings from the Intelligence Community*

During the spring and summer of 2001—what the 9/11 Commission later called the "summer of threat"—US intelligence agencies produced a number of increasingly dire threat reports, including the famous President's Daily Brief (PDB) that warned: "Bin Laden Determined to Strike in US." According to some experts, that report was a good piece of intelligence, though others found it to be shoddy.[38] In the end, none of the warnings specifically referred to the plot that became the 9/11 attacks, and US security services were unable to prevent the disaster.

According to some news accounts, US intelligence detected first indications of a novel disease outbreak in China as early as November 2019, even before Chinese authorities recognized or admitted the problem.[39] These reports have been denied by the National Center for Medical Intelligence, and we will probably need to wait for a national commission or congressional investigation before we know the full extent of early reporting on the virus by US intelligence agencies.[40] But current information suggests the traditional agencies of US intelligence reported on the new threat as soon as information became publicly available, although they were limited by a lack of specific knowledge in the early weeks. In January and February 2020, as reports of the virus began to multiply, intelligence agencies were warning about the rising threat. One official told the *Washington Post,* echoing the 9/11 Commission Report, that "the system was blinking red."[41] These warnings went to the White House and other executive branch agencies and were conveyed in a classified briefing submitted to the Senate and House intelligence committees in February.

The NCMI became seriously concerned about the virus by February 25, when it raised its warning level to what is called WATCHCON 1, the highest level of intelligence alert.[42] On February 27 an intelligence briefing to the Joint Chiefs of Staff stated the virus would "likely" become pandemic within next thirty days.[43]

We also have a general understanding of the reporting Trump was receiving in the early days of the outbreak. According to the *Washington Post*, Trump was briefed about the virus "more than a dozen" times in January and February, starting in early January.[44] The *Post* notes that these early reports were fragmentary "and did not address the prospects of a severe outbreak in the United States." A Trump administration official told *NBC News* that although the president's daily brief did contain more than a dozen mentions of COVID-19 in January and February, the briefings did not contain much more than was known in the public domain and did not contain warnings that the virus could spread around the globe.[45]

US officials have acknowledged that the first time Trump was briefed on the virus was January 23, when his briefer downplayed the threat.[46] Trump, who had a combative relationship with the intelligence community, later blamed his briefer for not having warned him adequately.[47] Although some experts have doubted whether such an exchange could actually have happened, according to the Office of the Director of National Intelligence Trump was indeed "told that the good news was the virus did not appear that deadly."[48] As many medical experts were realizing at that time, this assessment was badly flawed.

### Warnings from Disease Surveillance Systems and Other Open Sources

Regarding global pandemic threats such as COVID-19, the specific, tactical-level intelligence that can be most useful to head off a crisis is collected primarily from medical and public-health-surveillance systems. These systems were hampered by limited COVID-19 testing in the United States and many other countries, and reporting about the virus was blocked in China during the first weeks of the outbreak by local government bureaucracy and fears of upsetting officials in Beijing.[49]

The first English-language alerts about the new coronavirus came late on December 30, 2019, when HealthMap and ProMED issued reports about an unusual disease outbreak in Wuhan, China.[50] Other disease-warning systems began reporting about it on December 31, including the Canadian company BlueDot;[51] the Global Public Health Intelligence Network, that is also based in Canada;[52] and the website FluTrackers.[53] (See the appendix at the end of this book for a brief timeline of warnings and key events related to the outbreak.)

An Associated Press article from Beijing dated December 30 was one of the first reports in the US press to mention the outbreak.[54] The *South China Morning Post* from Hong Kong reported on January 1 about a new "mystery viral pneumonia outbreak" in Wuhan.[55] Helen Branswell, a reporter for the science and medical news website Stat, was one of the earliest to report on the outbreak, tweeting about the initial ProMED report on December 31 and then publishing an article on January 4 that warned the outbreak "might be caused by a new virus, and perhaps even a new coronavirus."[56] It was not until January 6 that the *New York Times* first reported on the mystery disease.[57] The first alert from the World Health Organization was on January 5.[58]

Elements of the US public health-intelligence system began watching the disease in early January and, according to DHS officials, the National Biosurveillance Integration Center began tracking the outbreak on January 2.[59] The first alert about the novel coronavirus from the CDC's Health Alert Network appears to have been on January 8, although CDC officials have said they had been alerted to initial reports of the virus as early as January 3 from discussions with colleagues in China.[60]

According to Reuters, the first word about the virus to reach the US national security system came on December 31, when an official at the National Security Council was forwarded an email from a Department of Health and Human Services attaché in Beijing about strange cases of pneumonia that had been detected.[61] But in the early weeks and even months of the crisis, US health experts were struggling with a lack of intelligence on the threat. We can see this struggle played out in what became known as the "Red Dawn" chain of emails exchanged by a group of infectious disease experts, who from January to March were sharing information about the virus. As the *New York Times* describes it, they were "grappling in the dark to understand what kind of threat was headed to American shores, and where it would land."[62] The emails show that in the third week of February concern turned to alarm among the experts, as they realized that the fight to keep the virus out of the country had been lost and it was time to turn to mitigation efforts such as closing schools and implementing lockdowns.[63]

One of the most important tools public health officials have in their arsenal is disease surveillance, which is designed to detect early indications of and monitor the spread of an outbreak. The COVID-19 pandemic revealed weaknesses in government disease-surveillance and -monitoring efforts. As one report notes, "Efforts to slow the spread of COVID-19 in the US have been stymied by the lack of an effective national surveillance system that can track the emergence of suspected and confirmed new cases in real-time."[64] Branswell, one of the first American journalists to recognize the significance of the outbreak, wrote on February 27 that "it's clear that the virus is spreading undetected in the United States—but how broadly it's spreading is an utter mystery."[65]

In order to be able to provide intelligence and warning, data must first be collected; but in the case of the pandemic, the US federal government did not have processes in place to ensure the collection of the data needed.[66] The first documented case of community transmission in the United States came not from an official government disease-surveillance program, but from a specimen collected February 24 by the Seattle Flu Study, which is funded by the Bill Gates Foundation.[67] Another example of the lack of government-monitoring capability is that the United States was revealed to have no single authoritative source for tracking the spread of disease. To fill that gap, Johns Hopkins University set up a COVID-19 dashboard that quickly became the national and international standard. As Jennifer Nuzzo writes, "The very fact that a university website, rather than the WHO, became the go-to source for information about the pandemic's spread exposed the gaping holes in international surveillance."[68]

A CDC report released in May 2020 states that limited community transmission of the virus likely had begun in the United States as early as late January and early February, at levels too low to be detected by the disease-surveillance systems being used.[69] As the *Washington Post* put it, "The virus was already circulating but at a level below the epidemiological radar."[70] Epidemiologists have called this a missed opportunity; for example, William Hanage from the Harvard T. H. Chan School of Public Health says, "Surveillance at the time was wholly inadequate to the task of catching a pandemic virus of this sort, whenever it was introduced."[71] Increased surveillance might have pointed to the need for greater testing earlier in the crisis, which could have helped to slow the speed of the outbreak.

Other studies have pointed to the importance of intensive surveillance and other interventions, such as testing in the early weeks of an outbreak—and not only in the United States.[72] For example, a report by Worobey et al. found that the virus strain that ended up infecting much of the United States did not actually enter the country until early February, meaning that "intensive testing and contact tracing could have prevented SARS-CoV-2 outbreaks from becoming established" in the United States and Europe.[73] Another report that reviewed the tools available for detecting COVID-19 notes, "The global spread of COVID-19 has been catalyzed by insufficient communication and underreporting," which could be addressed in the future by more aggressive surveillance systems, including smartphone surveillance.[74]

The failure of disease surveillance is closely linked to the widely noted failure of testing in the early weeks and months of the outbreak, because surveillance relies largely on the raw data provided by testing. Dr. Eric Schneider writes that "the United States has underfunded and undermined its disease surveillance programs."[75] Schneider complains that "our national disease-tracking effort seems stuck with well-meaning but scattershot efforts by tech companies using cellular phone signals, social media surveys, online searches, and smart thermometers as we try to guess where COVID-19 outbreaks may be lurking."[76]

Other evidence as well points to limitations in disease surveillance and detection that contributed to the severity of the pandemic. This is not a result of a lack of effort or will on the part of public health leaders, but it demonstrates an overall failure by US public health intelligence and surveillance. For example, the CDC announced in early February a plan for sentinel surveillance programs—targeted surveillance systems that provide early warning of outbreaks—in six cities, chosen because they already had well-established flu tracking programs. Dr. Nancy Messonnier of the CDC told a press briefing on February 14, 2020, that "results from this surveillance would be an early warning signal to trigger a change in our response strategy."[77] But in a number of those cities, such as Chicago and New York City, this surveillance effort was delayed and much less effective than it might have been.[78]

Other surveillance and tracking tools might have been useful, had they been tried. The CDC's Office of Advanced Molecular Detection uses genomic sequencing to track diseases, which means testing positive samples of a virus in order to detect new variants, but according to the *New York Times* it was slow to use these tools to track SARS-CoV-2.[79] The United States has been criticized for not conducting as much genomic surveillance as some other countries, although in response to the outbreak the CDC did create a consortium of more than one hundred labs and other institutions across the country, known as the SARS-Cov-2 Sequencing for Public Health Emergency Response, Epidemiology and Surveillance consortium, or SPHERES.[80] A related effort is the National SARS-CoV-2 Strain Surveillance (NS3) program to coordinate the work of public health laboratories across the country.[81]

Other disease-surveillance and -detection systems that might have been helpful in warning of the COVID-19 outbreak were either unavailable or unsuccessful. For instance, a US government program called PREDICT was begun in 2009 to search the world for viruses that could cross from animals to humans and cause pandemics. The funding for that program was cut off in September 2019, and although an emergency extension was announced in April 2020, the program was evidently not available to help accomplish its goal of prediction and warning in the case of COVID-19.[82]

In the early days of the pandemic the CDC used the Epidemic Information Exchange (Epi-X) system to send state officials emails about each arriving flight from China so they could track travelers for possible infection. But the data was time-consuming to process, such as in California, where according to some reports state officials received up to 146 emails per day, which they then had to forward to local health departments. Furthermore, the data had many errors, such as incorrect flight dates or times and other mistakes.[83]

An innovative surveillance tool that could have helped to track the early spread of the outbreak, had it been used widely and early, goes by the appropriate but unappealing name of sewage surveillance.[84] Wastewater surveillance, as it is also called, has been used in a number of countries around the world to watch for COVID-19.[85] As the outbreak spread in 2020, many US wastewater treatment plants also began testing their wastewater, but there was little coordination among the states or centralization of reporting.[86]

After coming into office, the Trump administration reduced the eyes and ears it had on the ground in China, where they could have served as open-source human intelligence reporters: it pulled more than thirty CDC staff members from its office in China and in 2019 eliminated funding for an epidemiologist embedded within the Chinese version of the CDC.[87]

One other kind of disease surveillance that has not been used effectively in the United States is contact tracing, which can help track and limit the spread of infection but has had only limited success in the United States.[88] Other countries such as Singapore, Australia, and South Korea have been more successful in minimizing infections in part through more widespread contact tracing, including digital tracing using cell phone apps, but these systems raise significant privacy concerns—part of the reason why they have been less successful in the United States.[89]

## Successes at the Local Level

The story of intelligence, warning, and COVID-19 is not one of complete failure, and several local communities in the United States experienced success. For example, sentinel surveillance was used successfully in Santa Clara County, California, where it helped to confirm community transmission in early March.[90] In Santa Clara the first case of community spread of COVID-19 was detected on February 27, and a sentinel surveillance program designed to test patients at four urgent care sites started on March 5. That testing finished on March 14, and found that 11 percent of tested patients were positive for the virus; within days officials in Santa Clara and five other Bay Area counties issued stay-at-home orders.[91] Santa Clara County's case shows both the importance of the speed of implementation of surveillance programs—if done in a few days or a week it can make a big difference in detecting and combating the spread of a virus—and, equally important, that surveillance efforts need to be linked to decision-making by policymakers.

Other examples of early and effective response to the outbreak include the Laguna Honda Hospital, a nursing home in San Francisco and the largest facility of its kind in California, which avoided the disastrous outcomes seen in other nursing centers during the pandemic. The city's mayor and public health director appealed for help from the state and the CDC, and within days received assistance from infection control experts, nurses, and epidemiologists, who worked with the facility's staff to implement protective measures, including strict quarantine for those infected, rigorous contact tracing to interview everyone who had come in contact with a sick person, and other tools to track the virus.[92]

The city of Seattle successfully used its already existing flu-surveillance system to detect the early signs of the outbreak.[93] At Travis Air Force Base in California, an early quarantine location for patients evacuated from China or coming off cruise ships, authorities activated a medical intelligence team, which collected and analyzed data to help military leaders make decisions before guidance was made available from national levels.[94] Guam had success in convincing the local population to sign up for a COVID tracing app, largely, it appears, because the population of the island learned early on about the seriousness of the virus when the USS *Theodore Roosevelt* was forced to dock there early in the crisis.[95]

## Assessing Tactical Intelligence and Warning

From what we know so far, the traditional US intelligence system failed to collect specific information on the spread and severity of the disease in time to enable decision-makers to act at the early stages of the COVID-19 pandemic. Part of the problem appears to be that prior to the outbreak, the IC had failed to focus sufficiently on the threat of infectious disease. A former senior intelligence official told the *Wall Street Journal* that units observing China, Russia, Iran, and North Korea got the most resources and attention, and "if those are one, two, three, four, this is 372" on the list of intelligence priorities.[96] Jim Himes, the second ranking Democrat on the House Intelligence Committee, said of US intelligence agencies: "They're not particularly designed to notice a cluster of symptoms in some far-flung corner of the world."[97] A House Intelligence Committee report in September 2020 that focused on US intelligence coverage of China also found that "the Intelligence Community places insufficient emphasis and focus on 'soft,' often interconnected long-term national security threats, such as infectious diseases of pandemic potential and climate change."[98]

To recognize the lack of expertise and focus on infectious disease within the traditional intelligence community is not to blame any individual analyst or official. But when the primary medical intelligence organization within the intelligence community—the NCMI—is a relatively obscure and low-level one, it is not surprising that any warnings it might issue are not likely to receive the necessary attention. A greater focus on health issues within the national security intelligence community might have led to greater clandestine collection on the virus as it spread in China in December 2019, which could in turn have produced more real-time, actionable intelligence on the growing threat and convinced leaders to take faster, stronger action against the threat.

Once the outbreak had been detected, the intelligence community was slow to understand how serious the situation would become, and its information appears to have lagged behind—or at best simply reflected—what was publicly available. Again, quoting a senior official's comments to the *Wall Street Journal* about intelligence reporting as of late January: "There was no assessment within the intelligence community that this was going to be a terrible pandemic."[99] Journalist and author Lawrence Wright puts it this way: "I wrote about 9/11 in *The Looming Tower* and I described the intelligence failure. Well, this was an intelligence failure. The US intelligence community had no idea about the catastrophic consequences that were about to enshroud our country."[100]

Until a national investigation is conducted, with full access to the classified record, we cannot know the full extent of what the intelligence community reported and when. But the extant public record suggests that the IC was unable to provide any warning about the outbreak beyond what was available through open sources such as ProMED. A cynic might wonder: Should the US taxpayer expect more from the roughly $85 billion spent on intelligence each year?[101]

It is, of course, impossible to know what early warning was available or what signals might have been missed. Perhaps there was simply nothing for the intelligence community to collect until the first clues about the outbreak began to be detected at the end of December 2019. It does appear, however, that signs existed, but the US intelligence community had not been listening. For example, the Chinese president's comments to Trump, as Trump relayed them to Bob Woodward, suggest that either signals intelligence or human intelligence could have detected early on the depth of concern about the virus on the part of Chinese leadership.

There have been reports that the US intelligence community was actually tracking the virus well before it was publicly identified, even in China—perhaps as early as November. So far those reports have been denied by intelligence community leaders. But what if that turns out to be the case? If a future commission or congressional investigation reveals that the IC had in fact been reporting on the outbreak well before it was recognized in open-source reporting, how would that change our assessment of intelligence failure? Certainly such revelations would alter significantly our understanding of how well US intelligence agencies performed in this crisis. Had the CIA in fact been reporting on the outbreak in early December, using human source reporting from within China, that would have been considered a significant success, as would early reporting by the National Security Agency (NSA) using signals intelligence, just to name one other example.

But the extensive public record of America's response to COVID-19 strongly suggests that such revelations would not change one key point: traditional intelligence reporting was largely ineffective in helping the United States respond to the outbreak. That failure was largely due to the lack of receptivity on the part of Donald Trump and other key administration leaders (which will be examined in the next section). It was also due to the fact that any such insightful reporting—if it did exist—did not reach the government and public health leaders who needed it. The White House COVID-19 task force surely should have received any such early warning, but the public statements by Dr. Anthony Fauci in January, February, and early March do not suggest any particular concern about the impact the virus might have in the United States. On January 21, 2020, Fauci said in a television interview, "This is not a major threat for the people in the United States, and this is not something that the citizens of the United States right now should be worried about."[102] On February 17 he told *USA Today* that the danger to Americans was "just miniscule," and even as late as March 9 he advised Americans to continue to go on cruise ships.[103] Fauci was certainly not alone among experts who downplayed the danger in the early months of the pandemic, and to point out these statements is not to criticize him but to argue that had more dire warnings been available, they do not appear to have been shared with the leaders and experts charged with communicating the nature of the threat to the American people.[104]

The traditional intelligence community is only one part of the intelligence system designed to anticipate and detect health threats. How, then, to explain the lack of precise, timely intelligence from public health disease-surveillance systems in the early weeks and months of the outbreak? Much of the problem lies with the complex system of international medical and health surveillance, which relies largely on self-reporting by countries that may be inclined, for economic or other reasons, to minimize the inherent danger (see chapter 3). In the case of the pandemic, global reporting systems were hindered in the important early days by the limited information available from China.[105]

Part of the fault, however, does lie with the public health and medical communities, which were hesitant to warn too loudly about the virus in the early weeks and months, largely because past warnings had turned out to be overblown.[106] As communications consultant Peter Sandman has written, "In February and well into March, COVID-19 warnings from US public health professionals were few and far between, a comparative whisper. The shouted message was that the (current) risk was low."[107] This is very similar to the problem that intelligence agencies and officials often encounter.

More broadly, the failures of disease surveillance in January and February 2020 do not reflect a lack of effort or professionalism on the part of the medical and public health communities. Rather, those failures reflect another problem that would look familiar to traditional intelligence experts: many disease intelligence and surveillance systems in place in the United States and around the world are not designed to provide the kind of detailed, near-real-time warning that is needed, and they suffer from a lack of data that all intelligence systems require.

Another way to assess the performance of intelligence and warning is to ask, What would effective warning about COVID-19 have looked like? Former senior British intelligence official David Omand has considered that question, and he argues that warning needs to be much more than simply including a given threat in a report or a briefing:

An effective warning is a loud shout to senior leadership for attention[,] giving:
- A strong knowledge claim about a very worrying development
- An assessment of why it really matters if it happens to us
- Sufficient illustration of how current policies may fail, in order to drive home the message that action is needed now to avoid disaster.[108]

To Omand, "warnings are a powerful combination of professional intelligence and scientific assessments."[109] When measured against Omand's benchmark, the warnings provided by the US intelligence, medical, and public health systems fell far short of what was needed.

## UNRECEPTIVE DECISION-MAKERS

The third factor that led to disaster on 9/11 as well as in the pandemic was a lack of receptivity on the part of key policymakers toward the warnings they received. Just as President George W. Bush and other top officials such as Condoleezza Rice were unreceptive to warnings about Osama bin Laden and al Qaeda, Trump and his team were slow to respond to the rising threat of COVID-19.[110]

Trump's lack of receptivity toward intelligence appears to be partly a result of his long-standing disagreements with the intelligence community over many issues, including over the question of whether the virus originated in a laboratory in Wuhan, China.[111] The most significant evidence for his lack of receptivity to warnings about the outbreak comes from journalist Bob Woodward, who has shown that Trump knew early on that the virus was more deadly than he had been saying in public, even though he still declined to act. On February 7, 2020, Trump told Woodward he had spoken the previous day with Chinese president Xi Jinping, and when Woodward asked what the two leaders had talked about, he said: "We were talking mostly about the virus." He went on to tell Woodward, "You just breathe the air and that's how it's passed. And so that's a very tricky one. That's a very delicate one. It's also more deadly than even your strenuous flus."[112] Trump later defended his actions as merely presenting a positive, optimistic face to the country, but his comments to Woodward clearly indicate that he understood the gravity of the situation.

It is not clear that Trump gained his understanding of the threat from intelligence; his February 7 conversation with Woodward suggests he was repeating what he had learned from the Chinese leader. But by early February Trump had received warnings about COVID-19 from a number of sources, including his top advisors and the intelligence community. According to Woodward, during an intelligence briefing in the Oval Office on January 28, national security advisor Robert O'Brien told Trump, "This will be the biggest national security threat you face in your presidency." Deputy national security advisor Matthew Pottinger agreed, saying he had been in contact with sources in China, and the world faced an emergency on par with the flu pandemic of 1918.[113]

Although the story of the pandemic is still being written, what we know at this point strongly suggests that Trump's inaction will be long remembered and on a par with other infamous cases in which politically motivated behavior and neglect of intelligence led to calamity.[114] It does appear that this part of the failure played a greater role in the COVID-19 disaster than it did in 9/11, because Trump was much less receptive to warnings about the virus than President Bush was to warnings about bin Laden and al Qaeda.

But it is too simplistic—and perhaps too easy—to blame only Trump. When decision-makers fail to listen to intelligence, it is the duty of intelligence agencies and officials to work even harder to make the warnings clear; from what we know at this point, there is no evidence that this happened as the threat of COVID-19 loomed. Trump's failure to act does also not explain similar failures in many other countries, and it does not fully explain the lack of early, decisive action in many US states and communities—where many of the most important public health decisions are made—in the early period of the crisis.

More generally, the failure to grasp the seriousness of the crisis in the early stages was a wide failure of intelligence, warning, and receptivity throughout the United States and around the world. This broad-ranging failure to understand the gravity of a threat has been seen before. The 9/11 Commission noted that Congress shared the blame for years of inattention to the terrorism threat in the years leading up to 2001.[115] Similarly, in the years and decades before the COVID-19 pandemic, Congress received many of the warnings about health threats but does not appear to have tried to use its tools of oversight and funding to increase emphasis on the problem. Much as years of success in counterterrorism may have lulled many Americans into a false sense of security before 9/11, it is possible that America's reputation for pandemic preparedness might have had the effect of reducing some decision-makers' alarm in the early weeks and months of the pandemic. One local health official who had been part of the Red Dawn email chain tracking the progress of the virus said about the US being ranked number one in the Global Health Security Index in late 2019: "We may have taken false reassurance in that."[116]

### Would Another President Have Done Better?

Deciding where, or even whether, to place blame for the lack of response to COVID-19 requires that we consider the question: Would another president have done significantly better in the early weeks and months of the outbreak? Of course it is impossible to answer this question with any certainty, but this book argues that the evidence strongly suggests that even with a president other than Donald Trump, the United States would have suffered greatly from the virus, and a significant part of the reason was a failure of intelligence.

This view rests in part on the fact that although some medical experts were sounding the alarm about COVID-19 in January and early February 2020, until the third week of February 2020 there was a lack of solid scientific consensus on how serious the problem was. It is likely that until that point, any president would have acted much as Trump did.[117] Better, earlier, and more specific intelligence might have made a difference—but in the absence of that actionable intelligence, a different president would not have made significantly different decisions in the critical early weeks and months of the pandemic.[118]

A second argument relies on the public statements of then-presidential candidate Joe Biden and other prominent leaders during the early months of the outbreak. Until at least late February, much of the US media was reporting the optimistic statements of public health experts, including Anthony Fauci. Joe Biden published an op-ed in *USA Today* on January 27, 2020, that charged

Trump was "the worst possible person to lead our country through a global health challenge," and he spoke out about COVID-19 on the campaign trail in late January and February, mostly to criticize the Trump administration's response.[119] Biden did not offer any specific plan for combatting the virus, and he continued to hold in-person rallies into early March, holding his last rally on March 9.[120]

## WHAT DID WE MISS?

Several studies have claimed to have found evidence that the virus had been circulating in China earlier than was originally thought; if these studies are correct, this could suggest that there had been clues that public health or traditional intelligence collection missed. One study, for example, found that the virus may have been circulating in Wuhan as early as August 2019.[121] The authors analyzed satellite imagery of hospital parking lots and search queries of disease-related terms on the Chinese search engine Baidu, and found increasing levels of hospital traffic and search volume beginning in late summer and early fall 2019. That report received a good deal of media attention but had not been peer-reviewed and was criticized for its methodology.[122]

Other scholars have examined whether early clues could have been detected through analysis of Chinese media, internet search, and social media behavior. These studies suggest that the virus may have been present prior to December, and if confirmed this could change our understanding of how best to detect future outbreaks.[123] A number of retrospective studies have been done to examine what information might have been available early on about the outbreak in China, if only we had been watching. Several such studies examined Chinese social media posts, and analyzed Chinese influenza surveillance data and internet search data.[124] Analysts found that the use of such data could have provided warning earlier than was given by the Chinese government. Wenjun Wang and colleagues, for example, examined posts for key words, including "Feidan" (which means SARS), on WeChat, the most popular social media app in China, and on Baidu, the main Chinese internet search engine.[125] They found that an analysis of data from WeChat could have provided warning of the outbreak about two weeks before the Chinese local authorities' official announcement of the outbreak on December 31, 2019.

## LESSONS FROM OTHER COUNTRIES

Was the pandemic really a *global* intelligence failure, even though a number of countries were relatively successful in taking swift action to reduce the outbreak? Yes it was, in part because even countries that were more successful than others have still been greatly affected—in terms of lives lost and citizens infected and in terms of economic and social impact. This crisis was a global intelligence failure because it came from a threat that does not acknowledge national borders and against which we are all truly in it together.

The pandemic was an intelligence and warning failure in countries other than just the United States. In Canada the small medical intelligence unit within Canadian Forces Intelligence began reporting on the virus in January 2020, but it appears that these reports, much like US intelligence reporting, were ineffective in helping Canadian security and health agencies prepare for the pandemic that was to come.[126] One report in the "Defence Intelligence Daily" on January 16 noted that "the outbreak appears to be contained" and "significant disease spread outside of China is unlikely."[127]

The Global Public Health Intelligence Network system, which was designed in Canada to use artificial intelligence and big data to detect early signs of outbreaks, appears to have not been active during the months leading up to the pandemic.[128] GPHIN was largely shut down in May 2019, when the government pulled doctors and epidemiologists away from surveillance of international health threats and reassigned them to other domestic projects, such as monitoring the effects of vaping in Canada.[129]

A Canadian inspector general report found that when the first reports of the outbreak came in, the GPHIN system issued daily reports, with the first report sent on December 31, 2019, containing a link to an article describing the outbreak of unknown origin.[130] But GPHIN did not issue an alert about the outbreak, which likely would have attracted more attention and could have gone to a wider audience.[131] As the outbreak spread, the network continued to take a low-key approach to the threat, assessing that the virus would have a minimal impact on Canada if it were to reach the country—that is, until March 11, 2020, when the WHO declared the virus a global pandemic. The official Canadian government report on GPHIN found that surveillance had not been well coordinated in the four years before the COVID-19 outbreak, partly because a key position, the chief health surveillance officer, had been vacant since 2017 and was scheduled to be eliminated.[132] "This is an intelligence failure," said Canadian intelligence scholar Wesley Wark. "We didn't have the early warning we needed and we didn't have a system to deliver it."[133] Wark has also written: "Faced with a new and unprecedented coronavirus threat, the surveillance and warning system failed, resulting in costly delayed responses."[134]

Britain provides another example of how strategic warnings can be ineffective. Well before the COVID-19 outbreak, a pandemic has been seen as the number one threat in the UK's National Risk Assessment process. David Omand has written, "During my time as UK Intelligence and Security Coordinator after 9/11, a mutated flu pandemic occupied the top right-hand corner of the strategic notice risk matrix—of all the threats and risks, it posed the most lethal potential combination of impact and probability."[135] Yet, as British psychiatrist and epidemiologist Simon Wessely has commented, even though pandemics were considered the number one threat for years, it took an actual pandemic to convince people to take the threat seriously.[136]

Australian intelligence expert Patrick F. Walsh writes that although the ten agencies that make up Australia's intelligence community did contribute to the country's pandemic response, "there is a lot more that Australia's national security enterprise, using its vast collection and analytical capabilities, can do to assist public health colleagues."[137] Even China, which had developed a national disease reporting system after the SARS epidemic, saw its disease surveillance warning systems fail.[138]

But the pandemic also saw cases of success, as several countries around the world responded quickly and—at least in the early months—effectively followed warnings of the virus. A number of countries were able to use surveillance and intelligence-gathering methods to track and control the spread of the virus, such as through using cell phone data for contact tracing, which can notify individuals if they have come in close proximity to someone who has been infected.

Success stories, such as experienced by South Korea, Taiwan, Vietnam, and Germany, suggest that effective use of intelligence and warning does not require that a country have the most extensive intelligence system, but it does require a strong intelligence-policy relationship and leaders who are willing to act.[139] For example, Scott Dowell, an infectious disease specialist at the Gates Foundation, writes that countries that have done well have had "early, decisive action by their government leaders."[140]

As a Council on Foreign Relations task force has concluded, a common factor among many—but not all—countries that responded quickly to COVID-19 was direct experience with previous outbreaks.[141] One of the most prominent examples of a swift and successful response is South Korea, which began screening and quarantining travelers from Wuhan on January 3, long before any cases of the virus had been detected within the country. South Korea's quick response appears to have been largely due to the fact that it had become sensitive to the threat of disease through its past experiences with SARS in 2003 and MERS in 2015. The country also learned broader lessons about disaster management after the April 2014 Sewol Ferry disaster, when the government and the ferry operator had been criticized for slow and inadequate action.[142] In addition to extensive testing, South Korea made aggressive use of contact tracing to track infections, led by its Epidemic Intelligence Service, including using credit card transaction data, cell phone location information, and closed-circuit television footage.[143]

Another widely recognized success was Taiwan, which, like South Korea, had learned important lessons from SARS and had a highly regarded national disease-surveillance system in place.[144] It began inspecting travelers coming from Wuhan as early as December 31, the same day that its CDC detected social media posts in China about an outbreak of pneumonia of unknown cause in Wuhan.[145] Taiwan's use of open-source intelligence has been praised, and its vice president, a trained epidemiologist, was a frequent public face of the crisis response on Taiwanese media and the internet.[146] One aspect of the successful response was the activation on January 20 of a Central Epidemic Command Center, reporting to the minister of health and welfare, to coordinate the government's response to the crisis.[147] Other elements of Taiwan's success include intelligence-related factors such as close surveillance of people who had been infected, combined with widespread acceptance of the use of face masks and tight restrictions on who could enter the country, along with strict enforcement of quarantines for those who did arrive.[148]

While Taiwan succeeded in largely closing its borders but allowing its economy and society to continue functioning much like normal, New Zealand took the approach of imposing a severe lockdown. A common factor in most successful countries, however, was the use of contact tracing, usually combining in-person tracing with cell phone apps, such as in Vietnam.[149]

As a number of observers have noted, there was no single formula for success in containing the pandemic. Ed Yong puts it this way:

The countries that fared better against COVID19 didn't follow a universal playbook. Many used masks widely; New Zealand didn't. Many tested extensively; Japan didn't. Many had science-minded leaders who acted early; Hong Kong didn't—instead, a grassroots movement compensated for a lax government. Many were small islands; not large and continental Germany. Each nation succeeded because it did enough things right.[150]

## AN ALTERNATE SCENARIO

I maintain that the proliferation of the pandemic was largely the result of a global intelligence failure, which implies that a better outcome—an intelligence success—was possible and could have occurred. What would intelligence success have looked like? What kind of actionable intelligence could have been developed, but was not?

Attempting to answer such questions requires a counterfactual analysis. Counterfactuals have been used to examine other aspects of the pandemic, and some believe that had nonpharmaceutical interventions such as lockdowns and social distancing been implemented only a week or two earlier, we could have effectively reduced the spread of infection and saved thousands of lives in the United States alone.[151] (The following is the first known use of a counterfactual to examine the intelligence and warning aspects of the pandemic.[152])

To be useful, any counterfactual assessment must be based on realistic information; it would be of little use to imagine, for example, that the CIA could have had a spy deep within the Chinese government who would have reported on the outbreak and saved the day, especially since we still do not know as of this writing how widespread the virus was in China or how much the Chinese government knew at the time. Similarly, a counterfactual should not rely on magic technological bullets like disease-surveillance systems that do not exist. Instead, a credible counterfactual must rely on already demonstrated capabilities that could reasonably have been used earlier or in different ways to produce different outcomes.

Success would have required more focus on health threats by traditional intelligence agencies long before the crisis; more linkage between those agencies and the fields of medicine and public health; more planning for and experience with tools such as contact tracing; and more training and education of leaders at all levels of government on what kinds of intelligence they would be likely to see in a pandemic. Success would not have meant preventing the spread of the virus, because from what we know about COVID-19 at this point it appears to have been just about the perfect enemy: lethal enough to cause great harm but not so lethal as to burn itself out, plus able to be transmitted before any symptoms are present.[153] Success would instead mean lessening the impact—doing a better job of "flattening the curve," as was so often talked about during the early months of the pandemic. Successful, actionable intelligence would only have had to give a few weeks' additional time to prepare and react to have dramatically impacted results.

No additional strategic warnings would have been necessary, but the warnings that were available would have needed to stimulate the development of new and better collection and analysis tools, making use of existing capabilities in the areas of human intelligence, signals intelligence, and disease surveillance. In the United States it would have required a long-term effort, over the course of several presidential administrations. Both the national security and the public health intelligence communities would have been better prepared to produce the tactical intelligence and warning that decision-makers needed in the early weeks and months of the outbreak.

In this scenario, agencies in the United States and around the world would have taken seriously their own warnings about the danger of a future pandemic, and programs such as the US government's PREDICT and Canada's GPHIN would have been up and fully running in late 2019. The CDC would not have cut back on its liaison personnel in China. Greater collection of Chinese social media and internet search activity—undertaken openly by public health systems but also secretly by intelligence agencies—would have given US leaders a better understanding of the debates going on in China at the end of December about the seriousness of the outbreak.

We might have had even earlier warning from traditional intelligence agencies if indeed it turns out that the virus was spreading widely in China before December. The IC would not have reassured President Trump on January 23, 2020, that the virus was not that deadly; instead it would have provided him with the sort of tactical intelligence that presidents regularly receive, such as transcripts of conversations among Chinese leaders expressing concern about the virus. Then, when the Chinese president told Trump about the seriousness of the outbreak the next month, he might have been more ready and willing to act.

The many agencies of the US intelligence community would have done more than report what was publicly available. They would have led, rather than followed, the state of knowledge in the scientific community and in the rest of the world. It is possible—but this counterfactual does not rely on it—that agencies such as the CIA and the National Center for Medical Intelligence could have done even more to get inside the thinking of Chinese leaders in the early stages of the outbreak: if they had been able to better exploit human and technological sources, they might have been able to understand the severity of the crisis in China even before Chinese leaders did.[154]

Even in the absence of warning earlier than the end of December 2019—when word of the outbreak first reached the West—any warning available could have led to more timely threat assessments delivered to political leaders and other senior officials by mid to late January. As the Independent Panel for Pandemic Preparedness and Response argues, earlier warning and better information sharing could have prompted the WHO to move faster in declaring a Public Health Emergency of International Concern, as it ultimately did on January 30.[155] But even if the WHO had not acted more quickly, wide-ranging planning could have begun at the federal, state, and local levels in the United States long before that date. This would have involved operational efforts, such as a review of emergency stockpiles of personal protective equipment, ventilators, and field hospitals, and sparked more intensive intelligence- and information-gathering efforts about China and other countries in the Pacific region.

The key time period for intelligence was late January and very early February. In this scenario of success, intelligence, medical, and public health organizations would have by this time begun shouting very loudly—to use the language of David Omand—that the United States and the rest of the world needed to pay attention to what was happening, and they would have had the data to back up their calls for alarm. The most effective intelligence would have come from the worlds of medicine and public health. By late January

2020 disease-surveillance systems would have been recalibrated to watch for the spread of the virus. New tools and techniques that had not yet been used on a large scale, such as wastewater surveillance, would have been used in earnest. The CDC would have rolled out a national dashboard, meaning the US government would not have had to rely on a private institution (Johns Hopkins University) for such an essential function. And, in what would probably have been the most visible part of the intelligence effort in the United States, by late February or March 2020 most Americans would themselves have begun contributing to the nation's intelligence-collection system by participating in digital contact tracing. Downloading and routinely checking a contact-tracing app would have become as much a part of our lives as face masks and quarantining.

All of these could have speeded the response in the United States by at least a couple of weeks and possibly as much as a month. As it was, the consensus of medical experts did not coalesce around the importance of measures such as social distancing until about the third week of February, roughly the same amount of time it took for the US intelligence community to take the virus seriously: the NCMI didn't go to its highest alert level until February 25 and a brief on the likelihood of a pandemic didn't go to the Joint Chiefs of Staff until February 27. The subsequent critical responses from the US government did not come until the middle of March, when widespread lockdowns and other interventions had already became commonplace.

In this alternative scenario, improved intelligence collection in December and January would have helped the medical and scientific communities form a consensus view a few weeks earlier than they did, perhaps by early February. The combination of intelligence and scientific consensus would have persuaded many leaders—even if not President Trump—to begin taking extraordinary measures several weeks earlier than actually happened.

## CONCLUSION

The COVID-19 pandemic was a global intelligence failure—a failure remarkably similar to the failure to prevent the 9/11 attacks. In both cases there was plentiful long-term, strategic warning before the threat arose, but it did little to avert disaster. In both instances the tactical-level, near-real-time warning that might have enabled decision-makers to take effective action was too little, too late. Key leaders were unreceptive to warnings they did receive.

As we consider this history of warnings unheeded, it is tempting to arrive at the same depressing conclusion that generations of intelligence professionals and scholars have reached after examining similar failures ranging from Pearl Harbor to 9/11: no matter how often or how loudly intelligence officials and other experts warn, their warnings will always be incomplete and leaders will continue to make decisions based on their own flawed judgments. As Richard Betts argues in his classic article from 1978, intelligence failure is not only inevitable; it is natural.[156]

It certainly may be true that intelligence failure is inevitable, and even natural, in the same way that disasters inevitably happen. But the key point is that none of these are inevitable *tomorrow*—there are things that we can do to prepare for and even anticipate disasters, in the same way there are things we can do to reduce the frequency of intelligence failures and anticipate threats before it is too late. The lessons learned from the COVID-19 pandemic hold clues for how the United States and the rest of the world can do better against the next pandemic or other global health threats. These lessons can even help us better prepare for and anticipate other kinds of threats and disasters beyond pandemics. The next chapter examines those lessons learned and provides suggestions for actions that should be taken.

## NOTES

Parts of this chapter draw on my article "Warnings Unheeded, Again: What the Intelligence Lessons of 9/11 Tell Us about the Coronavirus Today."

1. Scott Ritter, "The Staggering Collapse of U.S. Intelligence on the Coronavirus," *American Conservative*, March 24, 2020, https://www.theamericanconservative .com/articles/the-staggering-collapse-of-u-s-intelligence-on-the-coronavirus/; Micah Zenko, "The Coronavirus Is the Worst Intelligence Failure in U.S. History," *Foreign Policy*, March 25, 2020, https://foreignpolicy.com/2020/03/25/coronavirus -worst-intelligence-failure-us-history-covid-19/. Mark Stout offers a somewhat less sensationalistic analysis in his "A Response to Micah Zenko," *H-Diplo Essay 224*, May 1, 2020, https://issforum.org/essays/PDF/E224.pdf.
2. Julian E. Barnes and Adam Goldman, "For Spy Agencies, Briefing Trump Is a Test of Holding His Attention," *New York Times*, May 21, 2020, https://www.nytimes.com /2020/05/21/us/politics/presidents-daily-brief-trump.html; Katie Rogers, "Trump Now Claims He Always Knew the Coronavirus Would Be a Pandemic," *New York Times*, March 17, 2020, https://www.nytimes.com/2020/03/17/us/politics/trump -coronavirus.html.
3. Dahl, *Intelligence and Surprise Attack*, 23.
4. Ella Torres, Josh Margolin, Christina Carrega, and William Mansell, "US Intel Believe China Hid Severity of Coronavirus Epidemic While Stockpiling Supplies," *ABC News*, May 2, 2020, https://abcnews.go.com/US/coronavirus-live-updates-us -surpasses-65000-covid-19/story?id=70467380.
5. Julian E. Barnes, "C.I.A. Hunts for Authentic Virus Totals in China, Dismissing Government Tallies," *New York Times*, April 2, 2020, https://www.nytimes.com /2020/04/02/us/politics/cia-coronavirus-china.html.
6. Julian E. Barnes and Michael Venutolo-Mantovani, "Race for Coronavirus Vaccine Pits Spy Against Spy," *New York Times*, September 5, 2020, https://www.nytimes .com/2020/09/05/us/politics/coronavirus-vaccine-espionage.html.

7. Chris Whipple, "Anticipating COVID-19: A View from the Intelligence Community," October 16, 2020, https://www.brookings.edu/events/anticipating-covid-19-a-view-from-the-intelligence-community/.

8. Whipple, *The Spymasters*, 322.

9. Calder Walton, "US Intelligence, the Coronavirus and the Age of Globalized Challenges," Centre for International Governance Innovation, August 24, 2020, https://www.cigionline.org/articles/us-intelligence-coronavirus-and-age-globalized-challenges; Stephen Slick, "Getting Smart on Pandemics: Intelligence in the Wake of COVID-19," https://warontherocks.com/2020/04/getting-smart-on-pandemics-intelligence-in-the-wake-of-covid-19/. See also Aki Peritz, "The Intelligence Community Got the Pandemic Right, Then Politicians Botched It," *Washington Post*, September 11, 2020, https://www.washingtonpost.com/outlook/2020/09/11/intelligence-community-covid-success/.

10. Gregory F. Treverton and Molly Jahn, "COVID-19: We Had the Warning But We Lacked the Leadership," *The Hill*, April 5, 2020, https://thehill.com/opinion/white-house/490404-covid-19-we-had-the-warning-but-we-lacked-the-leadership.

11. Wirtz, "COVID-19," 4.

12. James Wirtz has termed this the "first law of intelligence failure." Wirtz, "Responding to Surprise," 51.

13. George J. Tenet, Testimony Before the Senate Select Committee on Intelligence, February 6, 2002, cited in Dahl, *Intelligence and Surprise Attack*, 131.

14. Bill Gates, "The Next Outbreak?: We're Not Ready," https://www.ted.com/talks/bill_gates_the_next_outbreak_we_re_not_ready?language=en; CSIS Commission on Strengthening America's Health Security, "Ending the Cycle of Crisis and Complacency in U.S. Global Health Security," November 18, 2019, https://healthsecurity.csis.org/final-report/. For a useful list of such strategic warnings, see Burwell et al., "Improving Pandemic Preparedness," 18.

15. Garrett, "The Return of Infectious Disease"; Osterholm, "Preparing for the Next Pandemic."

16. Institute of Medicine, *Microbial Threats to Health*, 8–9.

17. Klain, "Confronting the Pandemic Threat."

18. Global Preparedness Monitoring Board, "A World at Risk."

19. Nuclear Threat Initiative, "Global Health Security Index," October 2019, 9, https://www.ghsindex.org/wp-content/uploads/2020/04/2019-Global-Health-Security-Index.pdf.

20. David E. Sanger, Eric Lipton, Eileen Sullivan, and Michael Crowler, "Before Virus Outbreak, a Cascade of Warnings Went Unheeded," *New York Times*, March 19, 2020, https://www.nytimes.com/2020/03/19/us/politics/trump-coronavirus-outbreak.html.

21. FEMA, "2019 National Threat and Hazard Identification and Risk Assessment (THIRA)," 21.

22. Nahal Toosi, Daniel Lippman, and Dan Diamond, "Before Trump's Inauguration, a Warning: 'The Worst Influenza Pandemic Since 1918,'" *Politico*, March 16, 2020, https://www.politico.com/news/2020/03/16/trump-inauguration-warning-scenario-pandemic-132797. For useful reviews of the recent history of pandemic wargames and simulations in the United States, see Amy Maxmen and Jeff Tollefson, "The Problem with Pandemic Planning," *Nature*, August 6, 2020; and Mark Perry, "America's Pandemic War Games Don't End Well," *Foreign Policy*,

April 1, 2020, https://foreignpolicy.com/2020/04/01/coronavirus-pandemic-war
-games-simulation-dark-winter/.

23. Davies et al., "Urban Outbreak 2019 Pandemic Response"; Hope Hodge Seck, "The
Naval War College Ran a Pandemic War Game in 2019; the Conclusions Were
Eerie," Military.com, April 1, 2020, https://www.military.com/daily-news/2020
/04/01/naval-war-college-ran-pandemic-war-game-2019-conclusions-were-eerie
.html.

24. Center for Health Security, "About the Event 201 Exercise," n.d., https://www
.centerforhealthsecurity.org/event201/about.

25. NIC, "The Global Infectious Disease Threat," 5.

26. For a review of these reports, see Paul Miller, "How the Intelligence Community
Predicted COVID-19," *The Dispatch*, March 26, 2020, https://thedispatch.com/p
/how-the-intelligence-community-predicted.

27. NIC, "Global Trends 2025," 75.

28. NIC, "Global Trends 2030," xi.

29. Clapper, "Worldwide Threat Assessment," 11.

30. Coats, "Worldwide Threat Assessment," 21.

31. John Walcott, "The Trump Administration Is Stalling an Intel Report That Warns
the U.S. Isn't Ready for a Global Pandemic," *Time*, March 9, 2020, https://time.com
/5799765/intelligence-report-pandemic-dangers/.

32. Simone McCarthy et al., "How Disease X, the Epidemic-in-Waiting, Erupted in
China," *South China Morning Post*, February 27, 2020, https://multimedia.scmp
.com/infographics/news/china/article/3052721/wuhan-killer/index.html.

33. Editorial Board, "The Pandemic Didn't Come Out of Nowhere: The U.S. Ignored
the Warnings," *Washington Post*, April 21, 2020, https://www.washingtonpost
.com/opinions/global-opinions/the-pandemic-didnt-come-out-of-nowhere-the
-us-ignored-the-warnings/2020/04/21/3bf37566-7db3-11ea-a3ee-13e1ae0a3571
_story.html.

34. Jeffrey Frankel, "Foreseeable Unforeseeables," *Project Syndicate*, March 27,
2020, https://www.belfercenter.org/publication/foreseeable-unforeseeables?utm
_source=SilverpopMailing&utm_medium=email&utm_campaign=BIN_2020-3
-30%20(1)&utm_content=&spMailingID=23073705&spUserID=MTI2ODM2
MDMxMDMS1&spJobID=1701699349&spReportId=MTcwMTY5OTM0OQS2.

35. On the Trump administration's disregard of expert and scientific advice, see, for
example, Crystal Watson, "Confronting the Coronavirus: Perspectives on the
COVID-19 Pandemic One Year Later," Testimony to U.S. House of Representatives
Committee on Homeland Security, February 24, 2021, https://homeland.house
.gov/imo/media/doc/Testimony-Watson.pdf. Although Trump and his inner cir-
cle were largely dismissive of science, the administration as a whole continued to
fund many important science programs and the success of Operation Warp Speed
in developing vaccines is an indication that valuable scientific work did continue.

36. For a discussion of why strategic intelligence tends to have only a limited influence
on policy, see Marrin, "Why Strategic Intelligence Analysis."

37. Dahl, *Intelligence and Surprise Attack*.

38. Mark Lowenthal describes the PDB as a "fairly pointed strategic warning," while
Joshua Rovner sees it as an example of good tactical warning. Lowenthal, "Towards
a Reasonable Standard for Analysis," 305; Joshua Rovner, "Why Intelligence Isn't to
Blame for 9/11," Audit of the Conventional Wisdom (MIT Center for International

Studies, November 2005), 1–2, https://cis.mit.edu/sites/default/files/images/Audit
_Rovner_WhyIntelligenceIsntToBlameFor911.pdf; Zegart, *Spying Blind*, 108.

39. Ken Dilanian, Robert Windrem, and Courtney Kube, "U.S. Spy Agencies Collected Raw Intelligence Hinting at Public Health Crisis in Wuhan, China, in
November," *NBC News*, April 9, 2020, https://www.nbcnews.com/politics
/national-security/u-s-spy-agencies-collected-raw-intel-hinting-public-health
-n1180646. For a similar report, see "US Alerted Israel, NATO to Disease Outbreak in China in November—TV Report," *Times of Israel*, April 16, 2020, https://
www.timesofisrael.com/us-alerted-israel-nato-to-disease-outbreak-in-china-in
-november-report/. See also Kahana, "Intelligence Against COVID-19."

40. Some experts accept as likely correct the claim that the NCMI was reporting on
the outbreak in late November, but at this writing it is too soon to know. See, for
example, Gradon and Moy, "COVID-19 Response."

41. Shane Harris et al., "U.S. Intelligence Reports from January and February
Warned About Likely Pandemic," *Washington Post*, March 20, 2020, https://www
.washingtonpost.com/national-security/us-intelligence-reports-from-january
-and-february-warned-about-a-likely-pandemic/2020/03/20/299d8cda-6ad5
-11ea-b5f1-a5a804158597_story.html?utm_campaign=wp_news_alert_revere&
utm_medium=email&utm_source=alert&wpisrc=al_news__alert-politics--alert
-national&wpmk=1.

42. Deb Reichmann, "Medical Intelligence Sleuths Tracked, Warned of New Virus,"
Associated Press, April 15, 2020, https://apnews.com/article/da45eec432d6ff4cc
9e0825531e454a6.

43. Jenni Fink and Naveed Jamali, "Defense Department Expects Coronavirus Will
'Likely' Become Global Pandemic in 30 Days, as Trump Strikes Serious Tone,"
*Newsweek*, March 1, 2020, https://www.newsweek.com/coronavirus-department
-defense-pandemic-30-days-1489876.

44. Greg Miller and Ellen Nakashima, "President's Intelligence Briefing Book Repeatedly
Cited Virus Threat," *Washington Post*, April 27, 2020, https://www.washingtonpost
.com/national-security/presidents-intelligence-briefing-book-repeatedly-cited
-virus-threat/2020/04/27/ca66949a-8885-11ea-ac8a-fe9b8088e101_story.html.

45. Ken Dilanian, Courtney Kube, and Carol E. Lee, "Trump Administration Asks
Intelligence Agencies to Find Out Whether China, WHO Hid Info on Coronavirus Pandemic," *NBC News*, April 29, 2020, https://www.nbcnews.com/politics
/national-security/trump-administration-asks-intelligence-agencies-find-out
-whether-china-who-n1194451.

46. Barnes and Goldman, "For Spy Agencies."

47. Barnes and Goldman, "For Spy Agencies."

48. Whipple, *The Spymasters*, 323; "Intelligence Officials Back Trump's Assertion
that They Downplayed the Virus Threat in January," *New York Times*, May 4, 2020,
https://www.nytimes.com/2020/05/04/us/coronavirus-live-updates.html.

49. Steven Lee Myers and Chris Buckley, "China Created a Fail-Safe System to Track
Contagions; It Failed," *New York Times*, March 29, 2020, https://www.nytimes.com
/2020/03/29/world/asia/coronavirus-china.html.

50. Matt O'Brien and Christina Larson, "Can AI Flag Disease Outbreaks Faster
than Humans?: Not Quite," Associated Press, February 19, 2020, https://apnews
.com/article/100fbb228c958f98d4c755b133112582; ProMED, "Undiagnosed
Pneumonia—China (Hubei): Request for Information," *ProMED Mail Post* (blog),
December 30, 2019, https://promedmail.org/promed-post/?id=6864153.

51. Jerry Bowles, "How Canadian AI Start-Up BlueDot Spotted Coronavirus Before Anyone Else Had a Clue," *Diginomica*, March 10, 2020, https://diginomica.com /how-canadian-ai-start-bluedot-spotted-coronavirus-anyone-else-had-clue. Although some reports said BlueDot was the first to alert on December 30, the company's website confirms that it sent its first alert on December 31. https:// bluedot.global/, accessed December 29, 2021.

52. Murray Brewster, "Inside Canada's Frayed Pandemic Early Warning System and Its COVID-19 Response," *CBC News*, April 22, 2020, https://www.cbc.ca/news /politics/covid19-pandemic-early-warning-1.5537925.

53. Paul Farhi, "How a Blogger in Florida Put Out an Early Warning About the Coronavirus Crisis," *Washington Post*, March 14, 2020, https://www.washingtonpost .com/lifestyle/media/the-first-reporter-in-the-western-world-to-spot-the -coronavirus-crisis-was-a-blogger-in-florida/2020/03/13/244f39e6-6476-11ea -acca-80c22bbee96f_story.html.

54. "China Investigates Respiratory Illness Outbreak Sickening 27," Associated Press, December 30, 2019, https://apnews.com/article/00c78d1974410d96fe031f67ed bd86ec.

55. Kristin Huang, "World Health Organisation In Touch with Beijing After Mystery Viral Pneumonia Outbreak," *South China Morning Post*, January 1, 2020, https:// www.scmp.com/news/china/politics/article/3044207/china-shuts-seafood -market-linked-mystery-viral-pneumonia.

56. Marc Tracy, "The Medical News Site that Saw the Coronavirus Coming Months Ago," *New York Times*, March 30, 2020, https://www.nytimes.com/2020/03/30 /business/media/stat-news-boston-coronavirus.html?action=click&module= News&pgtype=Homepage; Helen Branswell, "Experts Search for Answers in Limited Information About Mystery Pneumonia Outbreak in China," Stat News, January 4, 2020, https://www.statnews.com/2020/01/04/mystery-pneumonia -outbreak-china/.

57. Sui-Lee Wee and Vivian Wang, "China Grapples with Mystery Pneumonia-Like Illness," *New York Times*, January 6, 2020, https://www.nytimes.com/2020/01/06 /world/asia/china-SARS-pneumonialike.html.

58. WHO, "Pneumonia of Unknown Cause—China," January 5, 2020, https://www .who.int/csr/don/05-january-2020-pneumonia-of-unkown-cause-china/en/.

59. Ken Cuccinelli II, "The Federal Interagency Response to the Coronavirus and Preparing for Future Global Pandemics," US Senate Committee on Homeland Security and Governmental Affairs, March 5, 2020, https://www.hsgac.senate.gov/imo /media/doc/Testimony-Cuccinelli-2020-03-05.pdf.

60. CDC Health Alert Network, "Outbreak of Pneumonia of Unknown Etiology (PUE) in Wuhan, China," January 8, 2020, https://emergency.cdc.gov/han/han00424.asp.

61. Katherine Eban, "As Trump Administration Debated Travel Restrictions, Thousands Streamed In from China," Reuters, April 5, 2020, https://www.reuters.com /article/us-health-coronavirus-nsc/as-trump-administration-debated-travel -restrictions-thousands-streamed-in-from-china-idUSKBN21N0EJ.

62. David E. Sanger, "Analysis: Will Pandemic Make Trump Rethink National Security?," *New York Times*, April 15, 2020, https://www.nytimes.com/2020/04/15/us /politics/coronavirus-trump-national-security.html.

63. Eric Lipton, "The 'Red Dawn' Emails: 8 Key Exchanges of the Faltering Response to the Coronavirus," *New York Times*, April 11, 2020, https://www.nytimes.com/2020 /04/11/us/politics/coronavirus-red-dawn-emails-trump.html.

64. Scott Weingarten, Jonathan R. Slotkin, and Mike Alkire, "Building a Real-Time COVID-19 Early Warning System," *Harvard Business Review*, June 16, 2020, https://hbr.org/2020/06/building-a-real-time-covid-19-early-warning-system.

65. Helen Branswell, "A Single Coronavirus Case Exposes a Bigger Problem: The Scope of Undetected U.S. Spread Is Unknown," Stat News, February 27, 2020, https://www.statnews.com/2020/02/27/a-single-coronavirus-case-exposes-a-bigger-problem-the-scope-of-undetected-u-s-spread-is-unknown/.

66. Clowers, "COVID-19: Key Insights," 12.

67. Chu et al., "Early Detection of COVID-19."

68. Nuzzo, "To Stop a Pandemic," 41. See also Amy Maxmen, "Why the United States Is Having a Coronavirus Data Crisis," *Nature*, August 25, 2020, https://www.nature.com/articles/d41586-020-02478-z.

69. Jorden et al., "Evidence for Limited Early Spread."

70. Lena H. Sun and Joel Achenbach, "CDC Chief Defends Failure to Spot Early Coronavirus Spread in U.S.," *Washington Post*, May 29, 2020, https://www.washingtonpost.com/health/2020/05/29/cdc-chief-defends-failure-spot-early-coronavirus-spread-us/.

71. Sun and Achenbach, "CDC Chief Defends Failure."

72. Morgan et al., "Disease Surveillance."

73. Worobey et al., "The Emergence of SARS-CoV-2 in Europe and North America," 564.

74. Udugama et al., "Diagnosing COVID-19," 3829. For another survey of the epidemiological surveillance challenges presented by the coronavirus, see Ibrahim, "Epidemiologic Surveillance."

75. Schneider, "Failing the Test," 301.

76. Schneider, 301.

77. Lauren Sommer, "Why the Warning that Coronavirus Was On the Move in U.S. Cities Came So Late," *NPR Morning Edition*, April 24, 2020, https://www.npr.org/sections/health-shots/2020/04/24/842025982/why-the-warning-that-coronavirus-was-on-the-move-in-u-s-cities-came-so-late.

78. Sommer, "Why the Warning."

79. Carl Zimmer and Noah Weiland, "C.D.C. Announces $200 Million 'Down Payment' to Track Virus Variants," *New York Times*, February 17, 2021, https://www.nytimes.com/2021/02/17/health/coronavirus-variant-sequencing.html?searchResultPosition=1.

80. David Cyranoski, "Alarming COVID Variants Show Vital Role of Genomic Surveillance," *Nature*, January 15, 2021, https://www-nature-com.libproxy.nps.edu/articles/d41586-021-00065-4. See also Carl Zimmer, "U.S. Is Blind to Contagious New Virus Variant, Scientists Warn," *New York Times*, January 6, 2021, https://www.nytimes.com/2021/01/06/health/coronavirus-variant-tracking.html?action=click&module=Top%20Stories&pgtype=Homepage.

81. CDC, "Science Brief: Emerging SARS-CoV-2 Variants," January 28, 2021, https://www.cdc.gov/coronavirus/2019-ncov/more/science-and-research/scientific-brief-emerging-variants.html.

82. Emily Baumgaertner and James Rainey, "Trump Administration Ended Pandemic Early-Warning Program to Detect Coronaviruses," *Los Angeles Times*, April 2, 2020, https://www.latimes.com/science/story/2020-04-02/coronavirus-trump-pandemic-program-viruses-detection; Charles Schmidt, "Why the Coronavirus Slipped Past Disease Detectives," *Scientific American*, April 3, 2020, https://

www.scientificamerican.com/article/why-the-coronavirus-slipped-past-disease
-detectives/.

83. Eric Lipton, Abby Goodnough, Michael D. Shear, Megan Twohey, Apoorva Man-
davilli, Sheri Fink, and Mark Walker, "The C.D.C. Waited 'Its Entire Existence for
This Moment'; What Went Wrong?," *New York Times*, June 3, 2020, https://www
.nytimes.com/2020/06/03/us/cdc-coronavirus.html; Myers et al., "Identification
and Monitoring."

84. Lawrence Goodridge, "Sewage Surveillance: How Scientists Track and Identify
Diseases Like COVID-19 Before They Spread," *The Conversation*, October 26,
2020, https://theconversation.com/sewage-surveillance-how-scientists-track-and
-identify-diseases-like-covid-19-before-they-spread-148307. See also Kim Ting-
ley, "Watching What We Flush Could Help Keep a Pandemic Under Control," *New
York Times*, November 24, 2020, https://www.nytimes.com/2020/11/24/magazine
/coronavirus-sewage.html?action=click&module=RelatedLinks&pgtype=Article.

85. Keshaviah, Hu, and Marisa, "Developing a Flexible National Wastewater."

86. Christian Daughton, "Wastewater-Based Epidemiology: A 20-Year Journey
May Pay Off for COVID-19," Stat News, January 7, 2021, https://www.statnews
.com/2021/01/07/wastewater-based-epidemiology-20-year-journey-pay-off-for
-covid-19/.

87. Marisa Taylor, "Exclusive: U.S. Axed CDC Expert Job in China Months before
Virus Outbreak," Reuters, March 22, 2020, https://www.reuters.com/article
/us-health-coronavirus-china-cdc-exclusiv/exclusive-u-s-axed-cdc-expert-job-in
-china-months-before-virus-outbreak-idUSKBN21910S; Marisa Taylor, "Exclusive: U.S. Slashed CDC Staff Inside China Prior to Coronavirus Outbreak," Reuters,
March 25, 2020, https://www.reuters.com/article/us-health-coronavirus-china
-cdc-exclusiv/exclusive-u-s-slashed-cdc-staff-inside-china-prior-to-coronavirus
-outbreak-idUSKBN21C3N5.

88. Jennifer Steinhauer and Abby Goodnough, "Contact Tracing Is Failing in Many
States; Here's Why," *New York Times*, July 31, 2020, https://www.nytimes.com
/2020/07/31/health/covid-contact-tracing-tests.html?searchResultPosition=1.

89. See, for example, Michael Pisa, "COVID-19: Information Problems, and Digital
Surveillance," Center for Global Development, March 20, 2020, https://www.cgdev
.org/blog/covid-19-information-problems-and-digital-surveillance; and Clark,
Chiao, and Amirian, "Why Contact Tracing Efforts."

90. Zwald et al., "Rapid Sentinel Surveillance."

91. Zwald et al., "Rapid Sentinel Surveillance"; Sommer, "Why the Warning."

92. Sarah Ravani, "How SF's Laguna Honda Averted Coronavirus Disaster," *San Francisco Chronicle*, July 27, 2020, https://www.sfchronicle.com/bayarea/article/A
-deadly-coronavirus-outbreak-seemed-inevitable-15433148.php.

93. Chu et al., "Early Detection of COVID-19."

94. Migliore et al., "Medical Intelligence Team Lessons Learned."

95. I am grateful to Kayed Lakhia for bringing this case to my attention. Cat Ferguson, "While Mainland America Struggles with COVID Apps, Tiny Guam Has
Made Them Work," *MIT Technology Review*, November 30, 2020, https://www
.technologyreview.com/2020/11/30/1012732/us-guam-covid-alert-app-exposure
-notification/.

96. Michael R. Gordon and Warren P. Strobel, "Coronavirus Pandemic Stands to Force
Changes in U.S. Spy Services," *Wall Street Journal*, November 22, 2020, https://

www.wsj.com/articles/coronavirus-pandemic-stands-to-force-changes-in-u-s
-spy-services-11606041000.

97. Gordon and Strobel, "Coronavirus Pandemic."

98. US House Permanent Select Committee on Intelligence, "The China Deep Dive:
    A Report on the Intelligence Community's Capabilities and Competencies with
    Respect to the People's Republic of China," September 2020, 27, https://intelligence
    .house.gov/uploadedfiles/hpsci_china_deep_dive_redacted_summary_9.29.20.pdf.

99. Gordon and Strobel, "Coronavirus Pandemic."

100. Sean Illing, "'We Did the Worst Job in the World': Lawrence Wright on America's
    Botched COVID-19 Response," *Vox*, February 9, 2021, https://www.vox.com
    /coronavirus-covid19/22202738/covid-19-coronavirus-america-anniversary
    -lawrence-wright.

101. Federation of American Scientists, "Intelligence Budget Data," accessed December
    29, 2021, https://fas.org/irp/budget/.

102. Nickie Louise, "Did Public Health Officials Mislead US?," *Tech Startups*, April 12,
    2020, https://techstartups.com/2020/04/12/public-health-officials-mislead
    -us-coronavirus-not-major-threat-people-united-states-not-something-citizens
    -worried-dr-fauci-said-janu/.

103. Jayne O'Donnell, "Top Disease Official: Risk of Coronavirus in USA Is 'Miniscule';
    Skip Mask and Wash Hands," *USA Today*, February 17, 2020, https://www.usatoday
    .com/story/news/health/2020/02/17/nih-disease-official-anthony-fauci-risk-of
    -coronavirus-in-u-s-is-minuscule-skip-mask-and-wash-hands/4787209002/; "Dr.
    Fauci Cruise Ships," C-SPAN.org, April 14, 2020, https://www.c-span.org/video/
    ?c4868772/user-clip-dr-fauci-cruise-ships.

104. See Helen Branswell, "The Months of Magical Thinking: As the Coronavirus Swept
    Over China, Some Experts Were in Denial," Stat News, April 20, 2020, https://www
    .statnews.com/2020/04/20/the-months-of-magical-thinking-as-the-coronavirus
    -swept-over-china-some-experts-were-in-denial-about-what-was-to-come/.

105. Associated Press, "China Delayed Releasing Coronavirus Info, Frustrating WHO,"
    June 2, 2020, https://apnews.com/3c061794970661042b18d5aeaaed9fae.

106. Peter M. Sandman, "Public Health's Share of the Blame: US COVID-19 Risk
    Communication Failures," University of Minnesota Center for Infectious Dis-
    ease Research and Policy, August 24, 2020, https://www.cidrap.umn.edu/news
    -perspective/2020/08/commentary-public-healths-share-blame-us-covid-19-risk
    -communication.

107. Sandman, "Public Health's Share of the Blame."

108. David Omand, "Will the Intelligence Agencies Spot the Next Outbreak?," *The Arti-
    cle*, May 18, 2020, https://www.thearticle.com/will-the-intelligence-agencies-spot
    -the-next-outbreak.

109. Omand, "Will the Intelligence Agencies?."

110. Dahl, *Intelligence and Surprise Attack*, 156–57; Harris et al., "U.S. Intelligence
    Reports."

111. Zachary Cohen, Alex Marquardt, Kylie Atwood, and Jim Acosta, "Trump Contra-
    dicts U.S. Intel Community by Claiming He's Seen Evidence Coronavirus Orig-
    inated in Chinese Lab," *CNN*, May 1, 2020, https://www.cnn.com/2020/04/30
    /politics/trump-intelligence-community-china-coronavirus-origins/index.html.

112. Robert Costa and Philip Rucker, "Woodward Book: Trump Says He Knew Corona-
    virus Was 'Deadly' and Worse Than the Flu While Intentionally Misleading

Americans," *Washington Post*, September 9, 2020, https://www.washingtonpost
.com/politics/bob-woodward-rage-book-trump/2020/09/09/0368fe3c-efd2-11ea
-b4bc-3a2098fc73d4_story.html. See also Maggie Haberman, "Trump Admits
Downplaying the Virus Knowing It Was 'Deadly Stuff,'" *New York Times*, September 9, 2020, https://www.nytimes.com/2020/09/09/us/politics/woodward-trump
-book-virus.html.

113. Costa and Rucker, "Woodward Book." This conversation is also described in Lawrence Wright, "The Plague Year," *New Yorker*, December 28, 2020, https://www
.newyorker.com/magazine/2021/01/04/the-plague-year.

114. For other examples, see Bar-Joseph and Levy, "Conscious Action"; Bar-Joseph and
McDermott, *Intelligence Successes and Failure*.

115. 9/11 Commission, *The 9/11 Commission Report*.

116. Jeffrey Duchin, cited in Matthew Mosk, Kaitlyn Folmer, and Josh Margolin, "As
Coronavirus Threatened Invasion, a New 'Red Dawn' Team Tried to Save America,"
*ABC News*, July 28, 2020, https://abcnews.go.com/Health/coronavirus-threatened
-invasion-red-dawn-team-save-america/story?id=72000727.

117. For example of some of the warnings, see Poland, "Another Coronavirus, Another
Epidemic, Another Warning." On the development of a consensus in late February, see, for example, Eric Lipton, David E. Sanger, Maggie Haberman, Michael D.
Shear, Mark Mazzetti, and Julian E. Barnes, "He Could Have Seen What Was Coming: Behind Trump's Failure on the Virus," *New York Times*, April 11, 2020, https://
www.nytimes.com/2020/04/11/us/politics/coronavirus-trump-response.html
?action=click&module=Spotlight&pgtype=Homepage.

118. Having a different president might have made a difference in the critical gap
between the third week of February, when a scientific consensus began to form on
seriousness of the problem, and mid-March, when the country as a whole finally
began to take the pandemic seriously. But even in the absence of better contact
tracing or other efforts, it is not at all clear that a different administration would
have acted much differently.

119. Joe Biden, "Trump Is Worst Possible Leader to Deal with Coronavirus Outbreak,"
*USA Today*, January 27, 2020, https://www.usatoday.com/story/opinion/2020
/01/27/coronavirus-donald-trump-made-us-less-prepared-joe-biden-column
/4581710002/.

120. Glenn Kessler, "How Specific Were Biden's Recommendations on the Coronavirus?," *Washington Post*, June 4, 2020, https://www.washingtonpost.com/politics
/2020/06/04/how-specific-were-bidens-recommendations-coronavirus/.

121. Elaine Okanyene Nsoesie, Benjamin Rader, Yiyao L. Barnoon, Lauren Goodwin,
and John S. Brownstein, "Analysis of Hospital Traffic and Search Engine Data in
Wuhan China Indicates Early Disease Activity in the Fall of 2019," Harvard Medical School, 2020, https://dash.harvard.edu/handle/1/42669767.

122. Hao Chen, Zi-Ming Du, Yu Kang, Zhenyu Lin, and William Ma, "Comment
on 'Analysis of Hospital Traffic and Search Engine Data in Wuhan China Indicates Early Disease Activity in the Fall of 2019' by Nsoesie et al.," 2020, https://
dash.harvard.edu/handle/1/42689379; Christopher Giles, Benjamin Strick, and
Wanyuan Song, "Coronavirus: Fact-Checking Claims It Might Have Started in
August 2019," *BBC*, June 15, 2020, https://www.bbc.com/news/world-asia-china
-53005768. For a more recent discussion of the virus's origins, see "More Evidence
that COVID-19 Started in a Market, Not a Laboratory," *The Economist*, March 5,

2022,  https://www.economist.com/science-and-technology/more-evidence-that
-covid-19-started-in-a-market-not-a-laboratory/21807945?utm_content=ed
-picks-article-link-1&etear=nl_special_1&utm_campaign=a.coronavirus-special
-edition&utm_medium=email.internal-newsletter.np&utm_source=salesforce
-marketing-cloud&utm_term=3/5/2022&utm_id=1069988.
123. Kpozehouen et al., "Using Open-Source Intelligence."
124. Dai and Wang, "Identifying the Outbreak Signal."
125. Li et al., "Retrospective Analysis"; Dai and Wang, "Identifying the Outbreak Signal"; Wang et al., "Using WeChat."
126. Murray Brewster, "Canadian Military Intelligence Unit Issued Warning About
Wuhan Outbreak Back in January," *CBC News*, April 10, 2020, https://www.cbc
.ca/news/politics/coronavirus-pandemic-covid-canadian-military-intelligence
-wuhan-1.5528381.
127. Wesley Wark, "Pandemic Warnings: Taking Stock of the Canadian Military's
Flawed Early Intelligence," Centre for International Governance Innovation,
October 27, 2021, https://www.cigionline.org/articles/pandemic-warnings-taking
-stock-of-the-canadian-militarys-flawed-early-intelligence/.
128. Grant Robertson, "'Without Early Warning You Can't Have Early Response': How
Canada's World-Class Pandemic Alert System Failed," *Globe and Mail*, July 25,
2020, https://www.theglobeandmail.com/canada/article-without-early-warning
-you-cant-have-early-response-how-canadas/.
129. Grant Robertson, "Health Minister Orders Review of Pandemic Warning System, Concerns Raised by Scientists," *Globe and Mail*, September 7, 2020, https://
www.theglobeandmail.com/canada/article-health-minister-orders-review-of
-pandemic-warning-system-concerns/. See also Lee and Piper, "Reviving the Role
of GPHIN in Global Epidemic Intelligence."
130. Auditor General of Canada, "COVID-19 Pandemic Report 8."
131. Adrian R. Levy and Wesley Wark, "The Pandemic Caught Canada Unawares: It
Was an Intelligence Failure," Centre for International Governance Innovation,
July 23, 2021, https://www.cigionline.org/articles/the-pandemic-caught-canada
-unawares-it-was-an-intelligence-failure/.
132. GPHIN, "Independent Review Panel Final Report." See also Murray Brewster,
"Canada's Pandemic Warning System Was Understaffed and Unready When
COVID Hit, Review Finds," *CBC News*, July 12, 2021, https://www.cbc.ca/news
/politics/global-pandemic-early-warning-1.6098988.
133. Murray Brewster, "Canadian Military Intelligence Unit Issued Warning About
Wuhan Outbreak Back in January," CBC News, April 10, 2020, https://www.cbc
.ca/news/politics/coronavirus-pandemic-covid-canadian-military-intelligence
-wuhan-1.5528381.
134. Wesley Wark, "The System Was Not Blinking Red: Intelligence, Early Warning
and Risk Assessment in a Pandemic Crisis," Centre for International Governance
Innovation, August 24, 2020, https://www.cigionline.org/articles/system-was-not
-blinking-red-intelligence-early-warning-and-risk-assessment-pandemic-crisis.
135. David Omand, "Will the Intelligence Agencies Spot the Next Outbreak?," *The Article*, May 18, 2020, https://www.thearticle.com/will-the-intelligence-agencies-spot
-the-next-outbreak.
136. Simon Wessely, "Transitioning to COVID-19's Next Phase: National Security Risks
and Opportunities Now," Strategic Multilayer Assessment webinar, April 13, 2021,

https://nsiteam.com/transitioning-to-covid-19s-next-phase-national-security
-risks-and-opportunities-now/.

137. Patrick F. Walsh, "Building a Better Pandemic and Health Security Intelligence Response in Australia," Centre for International Governance Innovation, August 24, 2020, https://www.cigionline.org/articles/building-better-pandemic
-and-health-security-intelligence-response-australia.

138. Myers and Buckley, "China Created a Fail-Safe System."

139. This section draws on COVID-19 research conducted by a number of organizations and researchers, such as: Exemplars in Global Health, https://ourworld
indata.org/identify-covid-exemplars; and Oxford Coronavirus Government Response Tracker, https://www.bsg.ox.ac.uk/research/research-projects/corona
virus-government-response-tracker.

140. Maxmen and Tollefson, "The Problem with Pandemic Planning," 29.

141. Burwell et al., "Improving Pandemic Preparedness," 26–27. On this point, see also Ferguson, *Doom*.

142. Kim, "South Korea's Fast Response."

143. Kim and Castro, "Spatiotemporal Pattern"; Ariadne Labs, "Emerging COVID-19 Success Story: South Korea Learned the Lessons of MERS," Our World in Data, June 30, 2020, https://ourworldindata.org/covid-exemplar-south-korea.

144. Fareed Zakaria, "What Sets Apart Countries that Successfully Handled the Pandemic?: Failure," *Washington Post*, September 17, 2020, https://www.washington
post.com/opinions/american-exceptionalism-has-become-a-hazard-to-our
-health/2020/09/17/9521a060-f921-11ea-be57-d00bb9bc632d_story.html; Jian et al., "Real-Time Surveillance."

145. Louise Watt, "Taiwan Says It Tried to Warn the World About Coronavirus; Here's What It Really Knew and When," *Time*, May 19, 2020, https://time.com/5826025
/taiwan-who-trump-coronavirus-covid19/.

146. Carmen Medina, "The IC Must Move Forward, Not Go Back," Cipher Brief, December 14, 2020, https://www.thecipherbrief.com/article/united-states/the-ic-must
-move-forward-not-go-back; Wang, Ng, and Brook, "Response to COVID-19."

147. Wang, Ng, and Brook, "Response to COVID-19."

148. Summers et al., "Potential Lessons"; Raymond Zhong, "How Taiwan Plans to Stay (Mostly) COVID-Free," *New York Times*, January 2, 2020, https://www
.nytimes.com/2021/01/02/world/asia/taiwan-coronavirus-health-minister.html
?searchResultPosition=1.

149. Todd Pollack et al., "Emerging COVID-19 Success Story: Vietnam's Commitment to Containment," Exemplars in Global Health, 2020, https://www.exemplars
.health/emerging-topics/epidemic-preparedness-and-response/covid-19/vietnam.

150. Ed Yong, "How the Pandemic Defeated America," *Atlantic*, September 2020, https://www.theatlantic.com/magazine/archive/2020/09/coronavirus-american
-failure/614191/.

151. Pei, Kandula, and Shaman, "Differential Effects of Intervention Timing."

152. I am grateful to Wesley Wark for his discussions with me about counterfactual scenarios.

153. Nicholas Christakis, "Nicholas Christakis on Fighting COVID-19 by Truly Understanding the Virus," *The Economist*, August 10, 2020, https://www.economist
.com/by-invitation/2020/08/10/nicholas-christakis-on-fighting-covid-19-by
-truly-understanding-the-virus?fsrc=newsletter&utm_campaign=the-economist

-today&utm_medium=newsletter&utm_source=salesforce-marketing-cloud& utm_term=2020-08-12&utm_content=article-link-6.

154. Scott Gottlieb, "Intelligence Agencies Can Help Stop Future Pandemics; Here's How," *Washington Post*, September 17, 2021, https://www.washingtonpost .com/outlook/intelligence-agencies-pandemic-prevention-gottlieb/2021/09/16 /079e7b78-164e-11ec-b976-f4a43b740aeb_story.html.

155. Singh et al., "How an Outbreak Became a Pandemic," 2118.

156. Betts, "Analysis, War, and Decision."

# FIVE

## Intelligence and Warning for the Future

Numerous medical experts today warn that another global pandemic is likely, whether from another novel virus such as the one that causes COVID-19, a variant of the flu or other infectious disease, or even a biological terrorist attack. What should be done to prepare for the next crisis to come?

Our future actions must be guided by the lessons learned from this latest pandemic as well as the lessons from previous disasters and intelligence failures. The primary problem for intelligence in the case of the coronavirus, as it was with the 9/11 attacks, was not a lack of long-term, strategic warning, since we know that intelligence agencies, health professionals, and other experts had been warning for years about the threat from an infectious disease. But the critical failures that must be addressed were twofold: first, the lack of timely, actionable intelligence on the threat as it developed; and second, a failure of receptivity toward intelligence on the part of policymakers that meant even timely warnings that did arrive were not heeded.

The preceding analysis does not imply that strategic warning is of no value. Warnings can help to place issues on the policy agenda and they can lead to planning that makes response more effective when a threat arises. Warnings can also be useful if they provide the impetus for intelligence agencies to develop new efforts to collect and analyze information and ultimately provide the tactical, real-time warning needed. But strategic warnings alone are rarely effective in preventing dangers from arising because they cannot get sufficient attention from policymakers who are too focused on current threats and challenges.

The importance of having timely, tactical intelligence on infectious disease outbreaks has been reinforced during the coronavirus pandemic. One of the key lessons is that the speed of response to an outbreak is critical; some studies have shown that acting more quickly—by even as little as one or two weeks—can have an immense impact on reducing deaths and minimizing the virus's spread.[1] One group of experts has argued, "The most urgent need for global public health is speed. With a viral epidemic, timing is nearly everything. The faster an outbreak is discovered, the better chance it can be stopped."[2]

For medical professionals this is not a new lesson. As one expert argued in an article written before the COVID-19 pandemic, "Even a single week of delay in recognizing an outbreak can have tremendous consequences for global health."[3] As an article in *Nature* put it, war games and simulations that preceded the pandemic taught that in an outbreak the actions needed to curb infection "must occur at hyperspeed."[4] The importance of timely tactical warning about almost anything is well understood by military and national security professionals: when a nation faces attack—whether from a hostile military or a terrorist plot—timely warning is critical. The coronavirus pandemic has demonstrated that the same principles of intelligence and warning apply when the threat comes from disease and the community at risk is not just a nation but the entire planet.

How, then, to develop the timely tactical intelligence needed for the next threat, and to ensure that when that intelligence is produced it will be heeded? The first step is to revamp our existing intelligence and early warning systems at the local, national, and international levels. Many of these changes will be difficult to achieve because they will require challenging traditional conceptions of what intelligence is and how it is organized around the globe and across the disparate communities of intelligence, medicine, and public health. The second step is to develop stronger connections between decision-makers and intelligence networks so that leaders are better able to understand and act on the warnings they receive. This is a difficult and recurring problem within the traditional realm of national security intelligence; to significantly improve intelligence-policy relations in the areas of health and medicine in the United States and around the world might be the most difficult challenge of all.

This chapter examines the changes that will be needed in American intelligence, starting with the traditional national security intelligence community and more broadly in the American national security system, as well as in the US medical and public health intelligence systems. Changes are also needed at the international level, first at the organizational and structural level and then to address the rising need for global disease warning systems. The vexing problem of intelligence receptivity must be addressed, and how to improve the state of intelligence-policy relations. The chapter concludes on a cautionary note, warning that as the United States and the rest of the world work to improve intelligence collection and analysis about disease threats, we must take care not to put into place systems that provide additional security but at the expense of a loss of civil liberties.

## CHANGES TO US INTELLIGENCE

Major institutional and cultural changes are needed to ensure the US intelligence community is better prepared to anticipate and prevent the next pandemic or other health disaster. One possibility might be to establish a new intelligence agency focused on health issues, but it seems unlikely that such an expensive undertaking will be approved.[5] A better approach would be to elevate the National Center for Medical Intelligence (NCMI) to the status of an independent national center reporting to the director of national intelligence. The NCMI would occupy a position comparable to the National Counterterrorism Center, established after the 9/11 attacks, and other national intelligence centers.

Several US allies are establishing new health intelligence organizations that could provide models for an enhanced NCMI. One is the new British Joint Biosecurity Centre, modeled on Britain's own counterterrorism center, the Joint Terrorism Analysis Centre.[6] The Canadian Public Health Agency has established a new intelligence branch intended to provide better warning of future pandemics.[7] A relatively inexpensive change that would help to raise the visibility and impact of the NCMI would be to appoint a more senior leader. The NCMI guiding instruction says that its director should be a flag officer or a member of the Senior Executive Service of the federal workforce, but that does not appear to have always been the case.[8] In April 2020, for example, Air Force colonel R. Shane Day was identified as the NCMI director when he denied that the center had reported on the coronavirus in November 2019.[9]

Beyond the elevation of the NCMI, other important changes should be made to the US intelligence community. A useful step that would have both practical and symbolic significance would be for the Department of Health and Human Services, and in particular its Office of National Security, to become a member of the IC, as James Danoy has suggested.[10]

In addition, a senior intelligence official should be appointed to oversee the IC's effort on health issues. Although the director of the NCMI might logically be expected to serve in that role, agency heads typically must devote much of their time to leading their large organizations; another national-level official is needed to oversee the coordination of health intelligence collection and analysis across the community. There are a variety of ways such a senior intelligence official could be named. Already existing are national intelligence officers (NIOs), who are senior experts on regional or topical issues serving on the National Intelligence Council who coordinate strategic and estimative intelligence analysis; national intelligence managers (NIMs) are the substantive experts within the Office of the Director of National Intelligence who coordinate intelligence collection and analysis in support of policymakers and other consumers of intelligence. Although appointing a senior health intelligence official as either an NIM or NIO would be useful, the most logical move would be to appoint a national intelligence manager dedicated to health security intelligence, while at the same time reinstating the position of national intelligence officer for warning (NIO/W).[11]

The NIO/W was abolished several years ago, when the intelligence community moved from a specialized warning system to an approach that has been termed "every analyst is a warning analyst."[12] In practice this change has meant that no one is responsible for warning, and the role of warning within the IC has been diminished.[13] An NIO/W is especially needed today, when the United States and the rest of the world face so many important strategic challenges.

Beyond organizational changes, the IC needs to develop new tools for forecasting and tracking health threats. The Intelligence Advanced Research Projects Activity (IARPA) is already working on this problem, and early in the pandemic it issued a call for research proposals to help anticipate and respond to pandemics.[14] The IC will also need to hire and train new health experts. Though the major agencies of the US intelligence community have long employed medical and scientific experts, they will now need to increase that focus and add experts in fields such as public health and epidemiology.[15] The US intelligence community has a mechanism for prioritizing issues and problems, called the National Intelligence Priorities Framework (NIPF), and that tool should be used to ensure that health issues are given sufficient priority.[16]

Although US intelligence agencies will need to acquire greater expertise in the area of medical intelligence, they should focus their efforts on the areas where they already have a comparative advantage over open-source medical intelligence; that would include, especially, on collecting and analyzing (often at a classified level) information about how other countries are responding to a threat. Such clandestine reporting is often critical for developing the actionable intelligence leaders need to guide their decisions. As an example of how this applies against a threat such as the coronavirus, reports in 2020 indicated that the intelligence community had for some time been warning that Chinese authorities were understating the number of infections within China.[17] Such assessments are also critical concerning suspect open-source reporting that comes from Russia, North Korea, and other nations whose autocrats are likely to have both means and motive to mislead the world.

Another area where the national security intelligence community can contribute is in the search for the origins of COVID-19. This is ultimately a question for medical experts, and as of this writing the scientific community is still divided on whether the virus emerged naturally and jumped from animals to humans (the predominant theory, known as zoonotic transmission) or escaped from a Chinese research lab.[18] In the face of China's efforts to hinder international investigations into the disease's origins, the tools and capabilities of traditional intelligence agencies are likely to be necessary if the world will ever gain a full understanding of where the virus came from. IC assessments have so far been inconclusive on the question of the virus's origins, and in February 2022 the director of national intelligence wrote: "All agencies assess that two hypotheses are plausible explanations for the origin of COVID-19: natural exposure to an infected animal and a laboratory-associated incident."[19] But US intelligence has concluded that Chinese officials did not have advance knowledge of its existence before the outbreak in December 2019 and that the virus was not developed as a biological weapon.[20]

The increased emphasis on health security intelligence will require a shift in mindset for US intelligence professionals, because traditionally—although not always—the US intelligence community has focused on human-caused threats and the secret information, clandestinely gathered, about those threats. The tools used to understand adversary governments and human activity will still be needed, and intelligence agencies such as the CIA will still need to steal secrets. The NSA and NGA will still need to use technical tools to monitor communications or collect satellite imagery to determine whether foreign governments are being deceptive in the information they release about health threats or are truly attempting to control the spread of an outbreak.[21] But, as Greg Barbaccia writes, "Infections don't have phones to intercept or track and offices to bug. There are no compounds to photograph via satellite, there are no financial transactions to track, and there is no housekeeper to flip as a spy."[22]

The intelligence community will need to make much greater use of unclassified, open-source information than it currently does. As Glenn Gerstell and Michael Morell write, "Information about the economy, health, supply chains and other public activities is far more likely to come from open sources than clandestine ones."[23] This will also mean that the intelligence community will be playing a more public role than it has in the past; as Calder Walton suggests, "When it comes to threats to public safety, such as pandemics, it must be questioned whether it is sufficient for the US intelligence community simply to provide warnings to policymakers, at which point its duties are discharged."[24]

It does not mean, however, that the national security intelligence community should take over any of the responsibilities or authorities that rightly belong to the medical and public health communities. As Greg Fyffe writes, "Intelligence involves providing a service to the lead department, not attempting to replace it."[25] This relationship could be made clear by the DNI through the use of terminology more commonly used by the US military to identify the chain of command and the lines of responsibility. Specific organizations within the intelligence community, such as the enhanced NCMI, the CIA, and the DIA could be tasked with providing support to the Centers for Disease Control; under this arrangement the CDC would be what the US military calls a "supported command."[26]

## CHANGES TO THE US NATIONAL
## SECURITY SYSTEM

Other changes should be made to the US national security system beyond the intelligence community. The first step is a change in perspective: to recognize that health security is an integral part of national security. As Dr. Julie Gerberding has stated, "Preparing for tomorrow's pandemic requires a new health security doctrine."[27] A task force sponsored by the Council on Foreign Relations argues that we need to make pandemic preparedness a national security priority equal with national defense.[28]

Changes made by the Biden administration represent a good start toward establishing health security as a key aspect of the nation's security. In its first National Security Memorandum, issued on January 21, 2021, the administration declared its intention to exercise global leadership in the global fight against the coronavirus, and it set out plans for "modernizing global early warning and trigger systems" to both help detect and respond to biological threats and develop a plan to strengthen intelligence community capabilities concerning pandemics and other health threats.[29] Since then the Biden administration has published a number of other documents setting out its pandemic goals, including a two-hundred-page national strategy and another document called the Interim National Security Strategic Guidance, issued in March 2021, which promised to "rebuild and strengthen federal, state, and local preparedness to handle not just this pandemic, but also the next one."[30]

Another positive step by the Biden administration has been to reestablish the National Security Council's Directorate for Global Health Security and Biodefense, which had been folded into another larger office during the Trump administration.[31] The office was restored by executive order on January 20, 2021, with Elizabeth Cameron appointed as the senior director—the same position she held under President Obama.[32]

Besides all these measures, much more needs to be done, and it will cost money. The United States needs to invest more heavily in public health, both at home and abroad. In fiscal year 2020 the US spent $750 billion on the military but only $547 million for global health security threats.[33] As Ed Yong notes, the US spends only 2.5 percent of its healthcare budget on public health.[34]

In addition to supporting international health security efforts, the US government will need to maintain close bilateral relationships with countries around the world, including those that might otherwise be adversaries. As long-time US diplomat Nicholas Burns has said, "To prepare for the next pandemic, we will have to work with China."[35] Such close relationships in the medical arena are possible. For example, well before the thaw in US-Cuban relations during the Obama administration, the CDC had long been able to work closely with Cuban medical authorities.[36]

The Department of Defense will need to increase its focus on health security. As a report by the Center for Strategic and International Studies has argued, the DoD should make it clear in the next National Defense Strategy that infectious diseases are a national security threat.[37] The pandemic has reinforced the belief that the threat will come not only from naturally occurring diseases but also from biological threats arising from state actors and others, including terrorists.[38] Some experts have argued that the pandemic may encourage terrorist groups to explore the use of biological weapons.[39] In response, the DoD needs to increase its funding for biological warfare defense, including for what is called the Chemical and Biological Defense Program.[40] Other experts have suggested the US should coordinate with allies to establish a BioDefense Fusion Center, with the goal of improving disease surveillance and reporting.[41]

More broadly, as Daniel Gressang and James Wirtz have suggested, the US government should conduct a net assessment to examine the ability of both government and society to cope with the threat in the future—and such an assessment could be conducted by a new interagency "skunkworks" to explore future hazards and develop creative ways to address them.[42] Leon Fuerth and other experts have argued for some time that the US government needs to improve its ability to foresee and plan for new kinds of problems, which Fuerth calls anticipatory governance.[43] We need greater foresight, as Fuerth writes, which "is about the disciplined analysis of alternative futures."[44] A new skunkworks could help provide this kind of foresight, but we also need policymakers to pay attention to that foresight. Lars Brozus and colleagues have made the point that "motivating policymakers to pay attention to foresight and risk assessment requires more than additional facts or sophisticated expertise."[45]

Just as the 9/11 Commission argued that we needed to institutionalize the use of imagination, we must now institutionalize the use of foresight. Experts have recommended that the coronavirus crisis, like 9/11, was largely a failure of imagination.[46] But actually, as I have argued elsewhere, we had plenty of imagination before 9/11, and as demonstrated here, there was no lack of foresight before the pandemic. What we need is institutionalized linkage between foresight and policymaking.

## CHANGES TO US MEDICAL AND PUBLIC HEALTH INTELLIGENCE

In addition to improving US national intelligence and security capabilities, we must work to improve medical intelligence and surveillance capabilities so that we can better detect and respond to future outbreaks. While US support is needed for improving international disease detection and response (discussed in the next section), much needs to be done within the United States as well.

The failure of the US medical and public health systems to effectively anticipate and track the spread of the coronavirus in the early weeks and months of the pandemic was something of a paradox. As Eric Schneider writes: "This country has generated many of the world's largest, most innovative, most profitable data companies. Yet when it comes to forecasting the spread of a major pandemic that is killing Americans and wreaking havoc on our economy, we seem oddly lost."[47] Part of the answer for next time will be to make better use of the tools and technologies that are already available. But significant changes will be needed in two areas: first, we must improve data collection; and second, we must improve the organizational structures involved with analyzing that data and turning it into intelligence.[48]

When it comes to collecting intelligence on disease threats, it is useful to keep in mind one of the truisms from the traditional intelligence world: in order to find something, it helps to know where to look. That is why intelligence agencies often use one kind of sensor to conduct a broad area search, looking for indications that the target of interest might be in that area. If those sensors are successful, then other kinds of more precisely focused sensors can be brought in to conduct a detailed search.

A broad area search—collecting data from as many sources as possible, covering as many potential threats as possible—can also help address another problem noted by traditional intelligence experts: the challenge of foreseeing an unfamiliar threat. Richard Posner wrote after the 9/11 attacks that "it is almost impossible to take effective action to prevent something that hasn't occurred previously."[49] Similarly, Jeffrey Shaman has said this about the effort to create an early warning system for new diseases: "I don't know of a field that has ever predicted something that had never existed before."[50] But it can be possible to detect a new or unexpected threat if intelligence and warning systems are set up to collect broadly. One example from public health of how early clues can come from unexpected sources was the outbreak of the West Nile virus in the United States in 1999: the first indication was the unexplained death of birds at the Bronx Zoo in New York City.[51]

One type of broad area search that may be useful is to use human waste as an early warning indicator of a new virus.[52] Sewage surveillance systems can test wastewater for the presence of the virus and, if it is detected in the wastewater from a particular community or neighborhood, residents could then be tested individually. This unconventional method is becoming more popular, and sewage surveillance is now being conducted in more than fifty nations.[53] The CDC is establishing a National Wastewater Surveillance System, and being able to use it to track the spread of the Omicron variant of COVID-19 in late 2021 demonstrated the utility of wastewater surveillance.[54]

Beyond the nontraditional approach of wastewater surveillance, a number of researchers have proposed new strategies and approaches for establishing a virus early warning system. Nicole Kogan and her fellow researchers, for example, developed a model that uses data from a variety of digital data streams to provide a near-real-time COVID-19 early warning system.[55] Others have suggested a different kind of warning and surveillance system that would link electronic health records from across the country through a real-time surveillance app that essentially automates syndromic surveillance reporting.[56] A report produced by the Duke Center for Health Policy proposed a nationwide COVID-19 surveillance system that would combine a number of different efforts and which would be coordinated by the CDC in collaboration with state and local public health agencies.[57] Such a system would require a robust capability for virus testing and contact tracing; an expanded system of syndromic surveillance; the use of serologic testing in order to understand past patterns of infection; and expansion of the capability to isolate and treat new cases, especially at the state and local level, and to rapidly implement contact tracing when outbreaks occur.

The collection of this data is only part of the challenge. Here again a lesson from traditional national security intelligence experience can be useful: in the face of a new (or newly recognized) national-level threat, it would be a good idea to set up a new national-level center or organization to analyze all the intelligence that is coming in. One of the major innovations following the 9/11 attacks was to establish the National Counterterrorism Center. In the wake of the COVID-19 pandemic, the United States needs not only a transformed National Center for Medical Intelligence (discussed earlier), but also a national center for public health intelligence. After the Ebola crisis, two public health experts suggested establishing such a center, and clearly it is needed now more than ever.[58]

At the US federal level, the National Weather Service offers a useful model for what could become a National Disease Forecasting Service. As Caitlin Rivers and Dylan George have described, until the 1960s weather forecasting in the United States was a decentralized effort involving academics and numerous government agencies that used a variety of technologies to track and anticipate the weather.[59] The establishment of the National Weather Service within the Department of Commerce proved to be a critical turning point that helped focus federal government efforts and gave weather experts what Rivers and George call "a permanent seat at the table" with policymakers.

Today, epidemiologists, public health specialists, and other experts need a seat at that same table. Rivers and George argue that the best way to do that would be through the establishment of a National Center for Epidemic Forecasting and Analytics (CEFA), modeled on the National Weather Center at the

University of Oklahoma.[60] Some experts caution that the problem of forecasting disease outbreaks is substantially different from forecasting the weather. Ricardo Castillo-Neyra has said, "Predictions are very good for weather forecasts. It's not that simple for infectious diseases. The number of variables is much greater."[61] But establishing such an office is an important first step, as is ensuring that it has access to senior decision-makers similar to the way the Scientific Advisory Group for Emergencies (SAGE) in the UK or the Infectious Diseases Modeling team in the Netherlands advise their governments. Other experts have also argued that setting up such an office is needed, along with employing other forecasting and analytics tools.[62] In a positive development, the Biden administration has established a Center for Forecasting and Outbreak Analytics, which could go a long way toward meeting this need.[63]

The pandemic has demonstrated the importance of local medical efforts, including surveillance and data collection.[64] In addition to new national-level efforts, new state and local systems will need to be developed to counter the threat of future outbreaks. As Eileen O'Connor of the Center for Homeland Defense and Security has suggested, we need to think in terms of "See something, Say something" for disease and health threats.[65] A local medical or public health official might be one of the first to notice some new outbreak or threat, and systems are needed that can enable that official to report what he or she has seen.

It may be even more important to establish state- or community-level warning systems so that those levels of government do not have to rely on federal direction—or in some cases, lack of direction. This is how military units, such as navy ships, are organized for intelligence support. Although ships typically operate as part of a larger battle group, each ship needs to be able to independently defend itself, which means that each needs access to intelligence and warning. Larger ships, such as aircraft carriers, have their own organic intelligence-collection and analysis systems, while smaller ships have direct links to other ships or shore stations that can provide them what they need. Similarly, in the United States larger cities, counties, and states need their own surveillance and warning systems, and smaller ones need access to that intelligence so they can make their own decisions about public health policy.[66] As Denis Nash and Elvin Geng argue, warnings about public health threats need to be made available to more than just local government and health leaders; actionable information about pandemics needs to be shared with "essentially everyone in society."[67]

## CHANGES AT THE INTERNATIONAL LEVEL

Changes must also be made to national and international medical-surveillance systems. The United States can do a great deal to promote international efforts, such as through increased support for international programs like the Global Health Security Agenda, which helps countries improve their epidemic detection-and-response capabilities. However, the most effective changes will be those developed multilaterally. As Council on Foreign Relations president Richard Haass has noted, "The pandemic is a textbook manifestation of globalization. What happened in Wuhan did not stay in Wuhan."[68] At the same time, Haass adds, "the response to this global crisis has been almost entirely national."[69]

## International Organizational Changes

Changes must be made to national and international medical-surveillance systems and organizations. A major problem is that the international system of pandemic warning and detection relies too heavily on the actions of individual governments, and the WHO does not have the clout to enforce existing requirements that nations monitor and report potentially serious outbreaks. One possible solution might be a new international treaty to provide the WHO with the authority to enforce reporting requirements.

A Council on Foreign Relations Task Force, for example, has argued that the International Health Regulations (IHR) that provide the WHO's legal framework could be revised in several different ways to encourage or even require states to report outbreaks promptly. The WHO could be required to notify all states whenever a state has not responded within twenty-four hours to a request to verify a potentially serious disease outbreak. Or states that fail to meet their obligations under the IHR could lose their voting privileges or be sanctioned in other ways.[70] Other experts have argued that the IHR needs to be strengthened, including with an inspection and monitoring system similar to the one used for enforcing nuclear nonproliferation treaties.[71] Johnathan Duff and colleagues have proposed an ambitious set of recommendations for a new global public health security convention.[72]

It seems unlikely that such measures will be accepted by the states that make up the World Health Assembly, which is the ultimate decision-making body for the WHO; and the WHO itself would be unlikely to exercise greater authority in any case, because it has a strong tendency to defer to its member states. The best that might be hoped for is for the WHO to convene what is known as an IHR Review Conference to examine how the IHR has been used in this crisis and seek improvements in information sharing.

A slightly different approach would be a global pandemic treaty, which has been called for by the European Council and supported by a number of national leaders and the director general of the WHO.[73] Experts have proposed that such a treaty could focus on reducing the risk of pathogens making the jump from animals to humans.[74] Swee Khor and David Heymann note that any global treaty needs to balance the need for a top-level body such as the WHO to set global standards and provide assistance, against the recognition that the most important efforts are taken at the individual state level, so any treaty must include incentives to encourage states to sign on to and follow it.[75] There is some good news here, as the World Health Assembly met in a special session at the end of November 2021 and agreed to begin a process of negotiations to create such a global pandemic treaty.[76] But this is only a very tentative first step—an agreement to talk at some point in the future.

If the coronavirus has taught us anything about the role of international organizations, it is that we cannot rely on the familiar agencies and models of the past. For example, beyond the much-criticized efforts of the WHO, the United Nations has been largely absent during the fight against the coronavirus. Although some experts argue the UN must continue to be included in future planning, the weakness of the global body was demonstrated when the secretary-general's call for a global ceasefire during the pandemic went largely unheeded.[77]

More broadly, the pandemic has upended traditional concepts of how global health is managed. As Sarah Dalglish has written, "The pandemic has given the lie to the notion that expertise is concentrated in, or at least best channeled by legacy powers and historically rich states."[78] Regional health organizations play a much more important role today than they did in the past, when the WHO was the clearly dominant institution governing global health.[79] New regional approaches are needed, involving both traditional organizations such as the G7, the G20, and European Union, and small states that may be better able than large states to serve as honest brokers or lead multilateral efforts.[80] Another useful idea is to establish a global Bio Force, which would involve a collaboration among national governments, international organizations, academic institutions, civil society groups, and private companies.[81]

## New Warning Systems

In addition to establishing new international institutions, a new global early warning system for infectious diseases and other health threats is needed to integrate the global hodgepodge of disease-surveillance systems that currently exists. Although many international disease-surveillance and warning systems are already in use, there is little coordination among them. As one report noted about existing disease-warning capabilities, "The current system suffers from fragmentation, a lack of coordination and collaboration, a need for sophisticated knowledge management, and virtually no sustained governmental and organizational commitment."[82]

Many experts have called for a better global warning system, with calls well before the coronavirus pandemic. After the Ebola outbreak in 2014, for example, Bill Gates provided the broad outline of a future global early warning system for disease.[83] More recently the Independent Panel for Pandemic Preparedness and Response (IPPPR) called on the WHO to establish "a new global system for surveillance based on full transparency."[84] Such a system will need to be able to detect and respond quickly to reports of outbreaks; one study, for example, suggests that a global target should be established such that every outbreak is identified within seven days of emergence.[85]

There are a number of different models upon which a global disease-warning system could be based. Some experts suggest we need a worldwide system similar to ones already in place that warn about earthquakes and tsunamis.[86] Another model could be the Famine Early Warning System Network, established in 1985 by the US Agency for International Development (USAID) to help provide early warning of food insecurity.[87] Leon Fuerth, the former administrator of USAID, has suggested establishing a Pandemic Early Warning System (PEWS) within USAID.[88]

Just as national security intelligence warning centers are designed to collect and integrate information from a wide variety of sources, a global disease-warning system will need to collect a wide range of data—ranging from commercial satellite imagery to social media posts to commercial sale transactions of pharmaceuticals—and produce near-real-time warning to national and local government and health leaders. Although such a global system is clearly needed, so far the pandemic has failed to inspire the sort of coordinated international effort that will be necessary. The good news is that a number of efforts are already underway or under discussion. The British government, for example, has proposed a global radar system to watch for outbreaks.[89] The WHO and Germany are establishing a pandemic warning hub based in Berlin and designed to improve on existing surveillance systems by connecting experts with new predictive tools, including artificial intelligence.[90]

Scientists are also working to develop a Global Immunological Observatory to provide early warning through serology: a global surveillance system that checks blood samples from around the world for the presence of antibodies, which would allow scientists to determine, in near real time, when communities have been infected by a particular virus.[91] The Biden administration is increasing efforts to use genomic surveillance to watch for new diseases in the United States.[92] Britain also uses genomic surveillance, and has set up a COVID-19 Genomics UK Consortium, which sequences 5–10 percent of positive samples throughout the country, looking for new and possibly more dangerous variants.[93] The importance of genomic surveillance was demonstrated in November 2021, when South Africa was able to use the technique to quickly identify the new Omicron variant of COVID-19.[94]

Another approach already in use is searching for new outbreaks and viruses in areas where animal-human disease spillover occurs.[95] There is a Global Early

Warning System (GLEWS) that monitors threats at the human-animal inter-face.[96] Another example is the Strategies to Prevent Spillover (STOP Spillover) Project, which aims to identify viral zoonotic diseases that migrate over into humans. This is a five-year program funded by USAID and led by researchers at Tufts University, which plans to work with ten high-risk countries in Africa and Asia to identify how viruses emerge and the sorts of human behaviors that can lead to outbreaks, such as eating the wild animals that present a significant spillover threat.[97] Efforts to look for new viruses involve intensive, often diffi-cult fieldwork at far-flung locations around the world.[98]

Other surveillance tools and intelligence-gathering efforts show promise for helping to detect and even prevent future pandemics. A number of studies have shown that increased monitoring of social media could have provided earlier warning of the COVID-19 outbreak, and scientists are examining ways to use tools such as epidemic modeling and artificial intelligence to predict future outbreaks.[99] Such big data–driven warning systems have significant limitations; as mentioned in chapter 3, systems such as Google Flu Trends have been unsuccessful in providing the near-real-time warning that will be needed to prevent future outbreaks from spreading.[100] But even if these tools are not a panacea, they can be the first step in tracking and anticipating the spread of disease. For example, researchers have been able to use cell phone data to predict the likely location of malaria outbreaks in Bangladesh.[101] This is why we need more projects like the Trinity Challenge, a bold effort to develop new and innovative tools and solutions to help the world prepare for the next major health emergency that is sponsored by a collection of business, academic, and philanthropic organizations.[102]

## IMPROVING RECEPTIVITY TOWARD INTELLIGENCE

As difficult as the task will be to develop new and strengthened international institutions and systems to provide warning of future pandemics, those alone will not be enough. New collection systems and cutting-edge technologies and tools alone will be insufficient for turning vast quantities of data into intelli-gence. To put it another way, it is not enough for intelligence to merely col-lect and connect the dots about current and future threats. It is a truism in the world of national security intelligence that intelligence and warning are of absolutely no use unless they spur the right person to take action, and this applies to health intelligence as well.

One of the most important intelligence lessons from the pandemic has been that unless decision-makers—both national or local—are willing to listen, warnings are ineffective. For example, the dysfunctional relationship between President Trump and the intelligence agencies and leaders who worked for him contributed to the failure of the US response in the early weeks and months of the COVID-19 pandemic. How can we ensure that leaders are receptive to the warnings they receive? Decision-makers should not automatically agree with intelligence assessments, but leaders must learn to trust their intelligence advisors and be willing to listen to the warnings they receive.

## Importance of Policymaker Receptivity

As seen in previous cases of intelligence failure, it is not enough for intelligence agencies, blue ribbon commissions, or other experts to warn of danger(s) coming—those warnings must be received by decision-makers who are willing to listen and then act. Even more recently, the January 6, 2021, assault on the US Capitol Building is another reminder that intelligence warning on its own is of little use if decision-makers are not receptive.[103]

How can we ensure leaders will listen to warnings? What makes them receptive? History shows there is no sure-fire way to make the system work, and in fact we do not want leaders to reflexively take action on every warning they receive. Sometimes a leader is receptive because of a personal interest in a topic or a threat. This is what happened to President Bill Clinton, who had read the Richard Preston thriller *The Cobra Event;* he became so concerned about the danger of biological warfare that he ordered intelligence assessments on it be undertaken, and funding for biodefense preparedness was increased fourfold.[104] President George W. Bush had a similar experience, becoming concerned about the pandemic threat after reading John Barry's book about the 1918 flu pandemic, *The Great Influenza.*[105] This kind of evolution in thinking occurs beyond health issues as well, perhaps most famously in the case of John F. Kennedy, who was influenced during the Cuban Missile Crisis by his reading of Barbara Tuchman's *The Guns of August.*[106]

Of course, we cannot rely on science fiction or the work of popular historians to grab the attention of decision-makers. But there is a validity to the point that leaders are more receptive toward threats that are more vivid or salient to them, often because they have experienced the threat personally. We often see this effect in terms of national security threats, such as in New York City in 1993, when the first bombing of the World Trade Center served as a focusing event that spurred officials in the FBI and the New York Police Department to increase attention and collection against international terrorism threats, ultimately foiling a planned series of bombings that could have caused a "day of terror."[107] We also saw this increased awareness during the pandemic: a common factor among many countries that responded quickly to COVID-19 was a direct experience with previous outbreaks.

There are other lessons in the traditional intelligence literature about policymaker receptivity that may be of benefit for medical and public health intelligence. Robert Jervis's work on the characteristics of policymaker receptivity is especially useful. Jervis has noted that "for intelligence to be welcomed and to have an impact, it must arrive at the right time, which is after leaders have become seized with the problem but before they have made up their minds."[108] This suggests policymakers may only be receptive to warnings at certain stages in the policy process. If you provide warning too early, before the policymaker is engaged with the problem, it may not resonate. If you warn too late, once the policymaker has made up his or her mind about the issue, then the warning is unlikely to change anything.

The most important factor associated with intelligence receptivity is the presence of a strong intelligence-policy relationship, and among countries that took swift action in response to warnings about the COVID-19 outbreak, such a relationship was often a factor. The key to having a strong intelligence-policy relationship is to develop it well ahead of time, so that when a threat arises the decision-maker trusts his or her intelligence advisors and understands the sources and methods involved in providing that warning.

The US military has long understood the importance of developing ties between intelligence and the leaders and operators (lower-level officers and commanders) it serves. For example, during the Cold War many aspiring naval intelligence officers—like me—got their start by undergoing basic training alongside aspiring pilots. Those pilots would later need to rely on the intelligence they received from their intelligence officers, and the navy knew that the best way to develop the needed trust between the two was to have them go through the same training regimen together: getting screamed at by the same drill instructors and freezing in the woods together. I wonder if the story of the pandemic would have been any different if, decades ago, Anthony Fauci and other leaders in the US public health system had gone through basic intelligence training alongside the future leaders of US intelligence agencies.

Another important factor in the intelligence-policy relationship is the establishment of effective communications. Ana Maria Lankford, Derrick Storzieri, and Joseph Fitsanakis argue that part of the problem during the COVID-19 pandemic was poor communication between the intelligence community and President Trump.[109] They offer useful suggestions, such as that intelligence agencies should do a better job of breaking out key warnings from among the day-to-day intelligence background. They recommend one change that is likely to be opposed by many traditionalists within the intelligence community, but which nonetheless deserves consideration: allowing intelligence professionals to offer policy advice to decision-makers in situations they believe involve catastrophic or even existential threats.[110] This concept is sometimes referred to in the US intelligence community as "opportunity analysis"; it is a means through which intelligence officials may identify specific intelligence gaps or opportunities that decision-makers might use to help advance their policy priorities.[111]

Even among intelligence professionals who support the idea of opportunity analysis, however, it is generally considered unacceptable for intelligence to offer specific policy advice. Mark Lowenthal, for example, describes the intelligence-policy relationship as a "semi-permeable membrane" through which policymakers can reach into the world of intelligence but which blocks intelligence officials from interfering with policy.[112] Today, however, when policymakers are faced with threats such as pandemics that cross the boundaries between traditional national security intelligence and medical intelligence, it seems clear that we must be prepared to let intelligence officials break through the traditional barriers that restrict them from offering advice.

The country's experience during the pandemic has also challenged another traditional intelligence taboo. Should intelligence have the job of persuasion? Consider: if intelligence officials believe some threat is significant but decision-makers do not appear to be listening, what should be done? If the problem at hand is a health threat such as a potential pandemic, is it appropriate for the traditional national security intelligence community to use its voice to encourage a leader to listen to the advice from medical and public health experts? The conventional wisdom among intelligence professionals is that this is not the job of the intelligence community. Certainly, if a significant threat or issue is identified, that importance should be conveyed appropriately. But by the conventional way of thinking, it is not the job of intelligence to determine which threats demand action. Only a decision-maker has the authority and responsibility to decide which threats are more serious than others.

This, too, is an outdated notion that needs to change. It is not up to intelligence officials to decide which threats deserve attention or which policies should be followed to address them. But experience has shown that threats are most effectively countered when the relationship between intelligence and policy is strong enough that intelligence officials are empowered to push back when they believe they are not being listened to on a matter of critical importance.

An example of how this can work comes from World War II in the Pacific theater during the months immediately after the Japanese attack on Pearl Harbor. Naval intelligence officials in Hawaii were watching for clues about what Japan's next move would be, and they began to see indications of a planned attack on the tiny island of Midway. Senior US leaders, including Adm. Chester Nimitz, doubted that the Japanese would target such an insignificant spot. Eventually the admiral's senior intelligence officer, Lt. Cdr. Edwin Layton, warned Nimitz about the growing evidence pointing toward Midway as the next target and implored him to visit the intelligence center to see the evidence personally. Nimitz, perhaps just wishing to move on to something else, told Layton he was too busy to visit the center but was willing to believe what Layton was telling him. Layton responded: "It isn't that. I want you to see it and be as convinced as I am."[113] Nimitz finally agreed to send one of his most trusted staff officers for a briefing, and after that officer became convinced, Nimitz was as well—ultimately contributing to the successful use of intelligence at the Battle of Midway.

It is nearly impossible for intelligence officials to be this persuasive unless they have already developed a close trusting relationship with the decision-maker. Even then, such an effort to convince a leader to pay attention can only be made rarely, since even the most understanding and receptive leader will simply stop paying attention. On rare occasions intelligence officials—whether from the traditional national security community or the worlds of medicine or public health—must have the opportunity to try to convince a leader to be as worried about a threat as they are.

### Leaders Must Be Ready to Lead

Although it is vital that decision-makers have a close enough relationship with their intelligence advisors that they are able to be receptive to the warnings they receive, a counterintuitive lesson from the pandemic is that leaders must not listen to experts—even intelligence experts—too much. Often in a complex crisis leaders must make decisions based on incomplete evidence from intelligence, from experts, and from science. This actually should not sound too surprising, because it is a standard understanding about military decision-making: leaders must be able to make decisions even when information is lacking. Mark Lowenthal, for example, has described an effective leader as someone who "can take decisive action in the face of incomplete, minimal, or even vastly discomforting intelligence."[114]

To support leaders who must make decisions under conditions of uncertainty, intelligence officials realize that their job is not to wait for hard scientific evidence. As the director of the National Center for Medical Intelligence has said, "We in the intelligence community love to be right, but we also know that in order to provide timely warning, warning in time for the customer to take action to mitigate what we've predicted, we have to be early."[115] This is similar to the argument made by the province of Ontario, Canada, during its inquiry after the SARS epidemic. The inquiry panel recommended the use of what it called the "precautionary principle": "action to reduce risk need not await scientific certainty."[116]

A number of experts have found that during the coronavirus pandemic, swift action was important, and leaders could not afford to wait for either intelligence certainty or scientific consensus. Waiting for experts to agree on the value of face masks, for example, led to unnecessary delays in providing the public with useful guidance. Researcher Ines Hassan and associates put it this way: "History has shown us that the risk of doing nothing while waiting for perfect data outweighs the risk of acting quickly with imperfect data."[117] Peter Sandman has made the similar point: "Officials should pay close attention to scientists, but they shouldn't give scientists their proxy."[118]

To some extent this is another area where the fields of medicine and public health can benefit from the lessons of national security intelligence. Military officers are trained to use and trust intelligence but also to know that ultimately the decisions—and the consequences—are their responsibility alone. Gemma Bowsher and Richard Sullivan likely have this lesson in mind when they argue that a science-led approach to COVID-19 led to failure, when decision-makers needed to make more use of the tools of intelligence, which are designed to operation under conditions of uncertainty and complexity.[119]

What should be done about this problem? It is far beyond the scope of this book to advise leaders on when they should or should not accept the advice of experts or go beyond the assessments of their intelligence advisors. But a good first step would be for leaders to recognize, as Danielle Allen has argued, that governance is not just a matter of "spitting out an answer" from scientists and economists—or from intelligence officials.[120] Governance is instead the task of integration and seeing the big picture in order to help society achieve the broader goals of government. Lawrence Freedman has observed the same lesson from the British experience with the coronavirus: scientists tend to wait for data, but policymakers should not and often cannot afford to wait. An example is the SAGE group in the UK, which waited for better data before recommending that strict lockdown measures be taken. As a result, the UK lost several days in late February and early March 2020, until a full lockdown was put in place on March 23.[121] Freedman has offered this advice about scientific expertise, which should apply equally to intelligence expertise: "Politicians should not be passive recipients of whatever expertise comes their way, but should rather engage with the experts to explore alternative options and their empirical foundations."[122]

## CAUTIONS ABOUT FUTURE SURVEILLANCE

One of the most important intelligence lessons from 9/11 came after that disaster had occurred, when US leaders gave intelligence agencies new, largely unchecked powers to monitor and surveil US citizens.[123] When these programs eventually came to light they caused a national scandal but also were found to have contributed little to increasing the country's security. The Bush administration's warrantless telephone monitoring program, for example, was a case study in what a democracy should not do. The lesson of the intelligence failure *after* 9/11 is that secret domestic surveillance programs are much more likely to fail than those begun with appropriate oversight and transparency.

Today many countries around the world are using cell phone tracking and other surveillance technologies to monitor those who have been infected or who are in quarantine after possible exposure. Although these tools have not been used as extensively in the United States as elsewhere, there are examples from the United States of successful contact-tracing programs. One lesson from these successes is that surveillance programs must be part of a broader effort to detect, track, and treat disease outbreaks. Colorado Mesa University in Grand Junction, Colorado, for example, has developed a holistic system that includes wastewater surveillance and testing in addition to tracing using a phone app.[124]

Such tools appear to be very useful, and in many countries and communities we can expect there will be pressure to institute some form of permanent "contact" tracing that relies on data from cell phones or other technologies to track and report on possible disease outbreaks. These systems raise a multitude of questions about privacy and civil liberties and in the United States in particular they have failed to be effective in stopping the spread of infection.[125] There has not been enough public discussion in the United States about whether such tactics should be used more widely. As computer scientist Susan Landau has written, "A robust public debate about the implications of deploying what is effectively a public surveillance system didn't occur; instead, many officials deployed these apps essentially overnight."[126]

If decisions are made to implement such surveillance programs, they should be implemented publicly and with full transparency and strong policies in place to protect civil liberties.[127] Any added security gained from these systems will need to be weighed against the loss to privacy or potential for abuse. The case of China provides an example of the lengths to which democratic governments do *not* want to go: it deployed an intrusive surveillance system that used facial recognition, contact tracing, and QR codes to track its citizens and in some cases to allow access to public areas to only those who were deemed free of disease. As Ashish Jha puts it, "It was as if the Centers for Disease Control and Prevention in the United States had used Facebook to track suspected COVID-19 patients and then quietly shared their user information with the local sheriff's office."[128]

A number of scholars and organizations have proposed recommendations for how privacy and data can be protected.[129] Others have proposed what are known as the Siracusa Principles to decide how to make the trade-offs necessary between protecting civil rights and obtaining security. These principles, developed by an international panel of lawyers, set out the circumstances when it may be appropriate for states to restrict citizens' rights.[130] Scholars such as

Simon Rushton and Nina Sun have argued that they can be used to determine when public health measures such as surveillance are appropriate.[131]

However, as Rose Bernard and teammates write, there is an inherent catch-22 in the use of intelligence and surveillance tools to detect disease outbreaks: to be effective such surveillance needs to be conducted continuously, even—or especially—when there is no outbreak present.[132] This kind of constant monitoring of the population raises tricky questions about civil liberties, ethics, and the law. Bernard argues that there must be restrictions on large-scale data collection of all kinds: "Both public health surveillance and nation state surveillance should be focused on outcomes or objectives: without a clear goal there is no justification for mass data collection."[133]

Many traditional intelligence professionals would resist such restrictions in the area of foreign and international intelligence collection. Certainly, intelligence agencies should have an objective or goal in sight, if only to justify the budgetary or other costs involved in conducting a collection program. But it is a truism in intelligence that more information (more data) is generally good, and the bar for justifying collecting intelligence in other countries is usually set quite low. When it comes to domestic surveillance, however, more data is not necessarily an achieved good if the collection process violates civil liberties without gaining sufficient benefit. It is clear that surveillance programs such as contact tracing should be treated as tools of medicine and public health and evaluated in the same way as the US Food and Drug Administration evaluates new medicines: before they are used on citizens they must be shown to be both safe *and* effective. In the context of public health, surveillance programs such as contact-tracing apps must be sufficiently *safe* for protecting civil liberties and personal freedoms but they also must be shown to be *effective* in preserving health and safety.

## CONCLUSION

If we are to stand any chance of anticipating and preventing even worse pandemics in the future, changes must be made in many places and at many different levels. The traditional US intelligence system will need to significantly increase its focus on nontraditional (i.e., health-related) threats, which will require both institutional and cultural change. The larger US national security system will also need to widen its focus; a good first step would be to conduct a net assessment to determine how best to improve the ability of the intelligence community and the rest of the national security establishment to anticipate future threats.

Even greater changes are needed in the areas of medical and public health intelligence and surveillance. The United States needs to consolidate its expertise and data-gathering systems under the auspices of a national center for public health intelligence, much as it formed the National Counterterrorism Center to bring together terrorism intelligence and expertise following 9/11. At the international level, the most important step will be to form a global pandemic warning system that integrates (but does not replace) the many different disease-surveillance and health-intelligence systems that already exist.

None of these efforts will be of much use, however, if decision-makers at all levels of government and throughout society are not trained and educated to be receptive toward the warnings that these systems and organizations produce. Leaders must be ready to lead, and that will sometimes mean being ready to act even in the face of contradictory intelligence or a lack of consensus among experts. If leaders do not have a strong and trusting relationship with the intelligence professionals and agencies who advise them, they will have little chance of using that intelligence effectively.

Leaders must also keep in mind that although better tools are clearly needed for disease surveillance, those tools often come at a price in terms of reduced civil liberties and the loss of personal freedoms. New surveillance systems should only be adopted or made permanent if they can be shown to be both safe for civil liberties and effective in keeping communities and individuals secure from diseases and other health threats.

There is, of course, no guarantee that intelligence—whether it comes from a national intelligence agency or from a local public-health-surveillance system—will be able to prevent a future pandemic or other health disaster. But if the steps outlined here are taken, we may find that when the next warnings of crisis come, they will be heeded.

## NOTES

1. Pei, Kandula, and Shaman, "Differential Effects of Intervention Timing"; Alagoz et al., "Impact of Timing."
2. Brilliant et al., "The Forever Virus," 90.
3. Hatfill, "Rapid Validation of Disease," 528.
4. Amy Maxmen and Jeff Tollefson, "The Problem with Pandemic Planning," *Nature*, August 6, 2020, 28.
5. This is the recommendation described in Shelton, "International Health."
6. Institute for Government, "Joint Biosecurity Centre," accessed December 30, 2021, https://www.instituteforgovernment.org.uk/explainers/joint-biosecurity-centre.
7. Murray Brewster, "Public Health Agency Launches Intelligence Team to Prepare for Future Pandemics," *CBC News*, June 24, 2021, https://www.cbc.ca/news/politics/phac-intelligence-pandemic-covid-1.6077639.
8. DoD, "National Center for Medical Intelligence (NCMI)," Instruction 6420.01 Change 3, effective September 8, 2020.

9. Ken Dilanian, Robert Windrem, and Courtney Kube, "U.S. Spy Agencies Collected Raw Intelligence Hinting at Public Health Crisis in Wuhan, China, in November," *NBC News*, April 9, 2020, https://www.nbcnews.com/politics/national-security/u -s-spy-agencies-collected-raw-intel-hinting-public-health-n1180646.

10. James Danoy, "Stopping the Spread: Pandemics, Warning, and the IC," NSI Law and Policy Paper, George Mason University, November 2020, https://nationalsecurity .gmu.edu/stopping-the-spread/.

11. Javed Ali discusses both options in "New Intelligence Steps to Address Infectious Disease Threats," *New America* (blog), May 4, 2020, https://www.newamerica.org /international-security/blog/new-intelligence-steps-address-infectious-disease -threats/.

12. Gentry and Gordon, *Strategic Warning Intelligence*, 85.

13. I am grateful to Roger Z. George for his comment on this point.

14. Ken Dilanian, "Coronavirus May Force the U.S. Intelligence Community to Rethink How It Does Its Job," *NBC News*, June 6, 2020, https://www.nbcnews.com/politics /national-security/coronavirus-may-force-u-s-intelligence-community-rethink -how-it-n1223811.

15. The CIA announced in October 2021 that it will establish the new Transnational and Technology Mission Center, designed to focus on both new technological threats and global challenges such as pandemics and climate change. This seems like a very broad remit for a single mission center, but nonetheless it is a positive step.

16. For information on the NIPF, see Office of the Director of National Intelligence, "Intelligence Community Directive 204."

17. Julian E. Barnes, "C.I.A. Hunts for Authentic Virus Totals in China, Dismissing Government Tallies," *New York Times*, April 2, 2020, https://www.nytimes.com /2020/04/02/us/politics/cia-coronavirus-china.html.

18. For a review of the scientific evidence supporting zoonotic transmission, see Holmes et al., "The Origins of SARS-CoV-2." A popular account of the debate is Carolyn Kormann, "The Mysterious Case of the COVID-19 Lab-Leak Theory," *New Yorker*, October 12, 2021, https://www.newyorker.com/science/elements/the -mysterious-case-of-the-covid-19-lab-leak-theory.

19. Director of National Intelligence, "Annual Threat Assessment February 2022," 19.

20. Director of National Intelligence, "Updated Assessment on COVID-19 Origins."

21. Calder Walton, "Spies Are Fighting a Shadow War Against the Coronavirus," *Foreign Policy*, April 3, 2020, https://foreignpolicy.com/2020/04/03/coronavirus -pandemic-intelligence-china-russia/.

22. Greg Barbaccia, "The Coronavirus Pandemic Will Force a Paradigm Shift in the U.S. Intelligence Community," *National Interest*, April 23, 2020, https:// nationalinterest.org/feature/coronavirus-pandemic-will-force-paradigm-shift-us -intelligence-community-147451.

23. Glenn S. Gerstell and Michael Morell, "Four Ways U.S. Intelligence Efforts Should Change in the Wake of the Coronavirus Pandemic," *Washington Post*, April 7, 2020, https://www.washingtonpost.com/opinions/2020/04/07/four-ways-us-intelligence -efforts-should-change-wake-coronavirus-pandemic/.

24. Calder Walton, "US Intelligence, the Coronavirus and the Age of Globalized Challenges," Centre for International Governance Innovation, August 24, 2020, https:// www.cigionline.org/articles/us-intelligence-coronavirus-and-age-globalized -challenges.

25. Greg Fyffe, "COVID-19 and Geopolitics: Security and Intelligence in a World Turned Upside Down," Centre for International Governance Innovation, August 24, 2020, https://www.cigionline.org/articles/covid-19-and-geopolitics-security-and-intelligence-world-turned-upside-down.

26. I am grateful to John Gentry for suggesting this idea. US military intelligence support arrangements are described in Joint Chiefs of Staff, "Joint and National Intelligence Support to Military Operations," July 5, 2017, https://www.jcs.mil/Portals/36/Documents/Doctrine/pubs/jp2_01_20170705v2.pdf.

27. Julie L. Gerberding, "COVID-19: Lessons Learned to Prepare for the Next Pandemic." Testimony to U.S. Senate Committee on Health, Education, Labor and Pensions, June 23, 2020, 4, https://www.help.senate.gov/imo/media/doc/Gerberding5.pdf.

28. Burwell et al., "Improving Pandemic Preparedness."

29. White House, "National Security Memorandum."

30. White House, "National Strategy for the COVID-19 Response"; White House, "Interim National Security Strategic Guidance," 16.

31. Glenn Kessler and Meg Kelly, "Was the White House Office for Global Pandemics Eliminated?," *Washington Post*, March 20, 2020, https://www.washingtonpost.com/politics/2020/03/20/was-white-house-office-global-pandemics-eliminated/.

32. White House, "Executive Order on Organizing"; Michael Crowley, "Announcing National Security Council Staff Appointees, Biden Restores the Office for Global Health Threats," *New York Times*, January 8, 2021, https://www.nytimes.com/2021/01/08/us/politics/announcing-national-security-council-staff-appointees-biden-restores-the-office-for-global-health-threats.html.

33. Burwell et al., "Improving Pandemic Preparedness," 53.

34. Ed Yong, "How the Pandemic Defeated America," *Atlantic*, September 2020, https://www.theatlantic.com/magazine/archive/2020/09/coronavirus-american-failure/614191/. For good recommendations about investing in public health, see Craven et al., "Not the Last Pandemic"; Bipartisan Policy Center, "Public Health Forward."

35. Shane Harris and Missy Ryan, "To Prepare for the Next Pandemic, the U.S. Needs to Change Its National Security Priorities, Experts Say," *Washington Post*, June 16, 2020, https://www.washingtonpost.com/national-security/to-prepare-for-the-next-pandemic-the-us-needs-to-change-its-national-security-priorities-experts-say/2020/06/16/b99807c0-aa9a-11ea-9063-e69bd6520940_story.html.

36. I am grateful to Dr. Jay Mercer for suggesting this point. See J. Stephen Morrison and Seth Gannon, "Health Cooperation in the New U.S.-Cuban Relationship," *Health Affairs* (blog), April 29, 2015, https://www.healthaffairs.org/do/10.1377/hblog20150429.047389/full/. On the potential for health cooperation with China, see Yanzhong Huang and Scott Kennedy, "Advancing U.S.-China Health Security Cooperation in an Era of Strategic Competition," Report of the CSIS Commission on Strengthening America's Health Security, December 2021, https://www.csis.org/analysis/advancing-us-china-health-security-cooperation-era-strategic-competition.

37. Thomas Cullison and J. Stephen Morrison, "What Has Covid-19 Taught Us about Strengthening the DOD's Global Health Security Capacities?" CSIS, May 11, 2021, https://www.csis.org/analysis/what-has-covid-19-taught-us-about-strengthening-dods-global-health-security-capacities.

38. Smith and Walsh, "Improving Health Security."

39. Pamela G. Faber et al., "Viral Extremism: COVID-19, Nontraditional Threats, and US Counterterrorism Policy," CNA, March 2021, https://www.cna.org/CNA_files

/PDF/IOP-2021-U-029346-Final.pdf; Lyon, "The COVID-19 Response." For a useful discussion of this threat, see Koblentz and Kiesel, "The COVID-19 Pandemic?."

40. Bill Beaver et al., "Key U.S. Initiatives for Addressing Biological Threats, Part 1: Bolstering the Chemical and Biological Defense Program," Council on Strategic Risks, April 9, 2021, https://councilonstrategicrisks.org/2021/04/09/briefer-key-u -s-initiatives-for-addressing-biological-threats-part-1/.

41. Michael Baker et al., "A Biodefense Fusion Center to Improve Disease Surveillance and Early Warnings to Enhance National Security," Security Nexus Perspectives, Asia-Pacific Center for Security Studies, September 2021, https://apcss.org/nexus _articles/a-biodefense-fusion-center-to-improve-disease-surveillance-and-early -warnings-to-enhance-national-security/.

42. Gressang and Wirtz, "Rethinking Warning."

43. Fuerth, "Operationalizing Anticipatory Governance."

44. Fuerth, 36.

45. Lars Brozus, "The Difficulty of Anticipating Global Challenges: The Lessons of COVID-19," IIGG Discussion Paper, Council on Foreign Relations, May 21, 2020, 8, https://www.cfr.org/sites/default/files/pdf/The%20Difficulty%20of%20Anticipating %20Global%20Challenges%2C%20The%20Lessons%20of%20COVID-19.pdf.

46. See, for example, the recommendations from experts compiled by the *New York Times* in "14 Lessons for the Next Pandemic," March 15, 2021, https://www.ny times.com/interactive/2021/03/15/science/lessons-for-the-next-pandemic.html ?action=click&module=Spotlight&pgtype=Homepage.

47. Schneider, "Failing the Test," 302.

48. On the need for better data, see Tarantola and Dasgupta, "COVID-19 Surveillance Data."

49. Richard A. Posner, "The 9/11 Report: A Dissent," *New York Times*, August 29, 2004, https://www.nytimes.com/2004/08/29/books/the-9-11-report-a-dissent.html.

50. Mark Johnson, "COVID-19's Toll Reveals Need for Fast Detection, Response; US Set to Begin Development of Outbreak Warning Systems," *Milwaukee Journal Sentinel*, April 12, 2021, https://infoweb-newsbank-com.libproxy.nps.edu/resources /doc/nb/news/181D040F8C32ECC0?p=AFNB.

51. Charatan, "Eight Die in Outbreak." I am grateful to Jennifer Hughes Large for suggesting this point.

52. Brady Dennis, "An Early Warning System for Coronavirus Infections Could Be Found in Your Toilet," *Washington Post*, May 1, 2020, https://www.washingtonpost .com/climate-environment/2020/05/01/coronavirus-sewage-wastewater/. Christa Leste-Lasserre, "Coronavirus found in Paris sewage points to early warning system," *Science*, April 21, 2020, https://www.sciencemag.org/news/2020/04 /coronavirus-found-paris-sewage-points-early-warning-system#.

53. Martin et al., "Tracking SARS-CoV-2 in Sewage." See also Emily Anthes, "From the Wastewater Drain, Solid Pandemic Data," *New York Times*, May 7, 2021, https://www.nytimes.com/2021/05/07/health/coronavirus-sewage.html?search ResultPosition=1; Freda Kreier, "The Myriad Ways Sewage Surveillance Is Helping Fight COVID Around the World," *Nature*, May 10, 2021, https://www.nature.com /articles/d41586-021-01234-1.

54. Keshaviah, Hu, and Marisa, "Developing a Flexible." See also CDC, "National Wastewater Surveillance System (NWSS)," accessed December 30, 2021, https:// www.cdc.gov/healthywater/surveillance/wastewater-surveillance/wastewater -surveillance.html; and Emily Anthes, "Omicron Is a Dress Rehearsal for the Next

Pandemic," *New York Times*, December 14, 2021, https://www.nytimes.com/2021/12/14/health/coronavirus-omicron-next-pandemic.html.

55. Kogan et al., "An Early Warning Approach."

56. Scott Weingarten, Jonathan R. Slotkin, and Mike Alkire, "Building a Real-Time Covid-19 Early Warning System," *Harvard Business Review*, June 16, 2020, https://hbr.org/2020/06/building-a-real-time-covid-19-early-warning-system.

57. McClellan et al., "A National COVID-19 Surveillance System."

58. Carney and Weber, "Public Health Intelligence."

59. Caitlin Rivers and Dylan George, "How to Forecast Outbreaks and Pandemics," *Foreign Affairs*, June 29, 2020, https://www.foreignaffairs.com/articles/united-states/2020-06-29/how-forecast-outbreaks-and-pandemics.

60. Rivers and George, "How to Forecast Outbreaks." See also Caitlin Rivers et al., "Modernizing and Expanding Outbreak Science to Support Better Decision Making During Public Health Crises: Lessons for COVID-19 and Beyond," Johns Hopkins Center for Health Security, March 24, 2020, https://www.centerforhealthsecurity.org/our-work/publications/modernizing-and-expanding-outbreak-science-to-support-better-decision-making-during-public-health-crises.

61. Johnson, "COVID's Toll Reveals Need for Fast Detection, Response."

62. Julia Ciocca et al., "How the U.S. Government Can Learn to See the Future," *Lawfare* (blog), May 9, 2021, https://www.lawfareblog.com/how-us-government-can-learn-see-future. See also Adam Rogers, "It's Time for a National Pandemic Protection Agency," *Wired*, February 3, 2021, https://www.wired.com/story/its-time-for-a-national-pandemic-prediction-agency/.

63. White House, "National Security Memorandum"; Jeneen Interlandi, "Inside the C.D.C.'s Pandemic 'Weather Service,'" *New York Times*, November 22, 2021, https://www.nytimes.com/2021/11/22/magazine/cdc-pandemic-prediction.html. The new center was announced as this book was being finished: CDC, "CDC Launches New Center for Forecasting and Outbreak Analytics," April 19, 2022, https://www.cdc.gov/media/releases/2022/p0419-forecasting-center.html.

64. Chu et al., "Early Detection."

65. Center for Homeland Defense and Security Executive Education Program, "What Comes Next?: Virus Variants, Vaccine Next Steps, and Preventing Future Pandemics," webinar, April 29, 2021.

66. I am grateful to Jay Mercer for suggesting the analogy to navy intelligence.

67. Nash and Geng, "Goal-Aligned, Epidemic Intelligence," 1156.

68. Burwell et al., "Improving Pandemic Preparedness," viii.

69. Burwell et al., ix.

70. Burwell et al., 90.

71. Taylor et al., "Solidarity"; Gostin, "The Coronavirus Pandemic."

72. Duff et al., "A Global Public Health Convention."

73. Consilium–European Union, "Statement of the Members of the European Council," SN2/21, February 26, 2021, https://www.consilium.europa.eu/media/48625/2526-02-21-euco-statement-en.pdf. On the idea of a global pandemic treaty, see also Lothar H Wieler, "Report of the Review Committee on the Functioning of the International Health Regulations (2005) during the COVID-19 Response," WHO, May 5, 2021, 50, https://cdn.who.int/media/docs/default-source/documents/emergencies/a74_9add1-en.pdf?sfvrsn=d5d22fdf_1&download=true; and Monti et al., "A New Strategy."

74. Vinuales et al., "A Global Pandemic Treaty."

75. Khor and Heymann, "Pandemic Preparedness."
76. Adam Taylor and Adela Suliman, "World Agrees to Negotiate a Global 'Pandemic Treaty' to Fight the Next Outbreak," *Washington Post*, December 1, 2021, https://www.washingtonpost.com/world/2021/12/01/who-coronavirus-pandemic-agreement-treaty/.
77. Suzanne Nossel, "The World Still Needs the UN," *Foreign Affairs*, March 18, 2021, https://www.foreignaffairs.com/articles/world/2021-03-18/world-still-needs-un?utm_medium=newsletters&utm_source=fabackstory&utm_content=20210509&utm_campaign=FA%20Backstory_050921_How%20to%20Rule%20the%20World&utm_term=fa-backstory-2019; Richard Gowan, "What's Happened to the UN Secretary-General's COVID-19 Ceasefire Call?," International Crisis Group, June 16, 2020, https://www.crisisgroup.org/global/whats-happened-un-secretary-generals-covid-19-ceasefire-call.
78. Dalglish, "COVID-19 Gives the Lie," 1189.
79. Jha, "System Failure."
80. Jared Cohen and Richard Fontaine, "The Case for Microlateralism: With U.S. Support, Small States Can Ably Lead Global Efforts," *Foreign Affairs*, April 29, 2021, https://www.foreignaffairs.com/articles/world/2021-04-29/case-microlateralism?utm_medium=newsletters&utm_source=fabackstory&utm_content=20210509&utm_campaign=FA%20Backstory_050921_How%20to%20Rule%20the%20World&utm_term=fa-backstory-2019.
81. "Francis DeSouza on the Need for a Global 'Bio Force' to Track Viruses," *The Economist*, February 9, 2021, https://www.economist.com/by-invitation/2021/02/09/francis-desouza-on-the-need-for-a-global-bio-force-to-track-viruses.
82. Esther Krofah, Carly Gasca, and Anna Degarmo, "A Global Early Warning System for Pandemics," Milken Institute, 2021, 2, https://milkeninstitute.org/sites/default/files/2021-06/A%20Global%20Early%20Warning%20System%20for%20Pandemics.pdf.
83. Gates, "The Next Epidemic."
84. IPPPR, "COVID-19," 53.
85. Frieden et al., "7-1-7."
86. Michael C. Lu, "Future Pandemics Can Be Prevented, But That'll Rely on Unprecedented Global Cooperation," *Washington Post*, April 17, 2020, https://www.washingtonpost.com/health/future-pandemics-can-be-prevented-but-thatll-rely-on-unprecedented-global-cooperation/2020/04/16/0caca7b8-7e6d-11ea-8013-1b6da0e4a2b7_story.html.
87. FEWS NET, "About us," accessed December 30, 2021, https://fews.net/about-us.
88. Andrew S. Natsios, "Predicting the Next Pandemic," *Foreign Affairs*, July 14, 2020, https://www.foreignaffairs.com/articles/united-states/2020-07-14/predicting-next-pandemic?utm_medium=newsletters&utm_source=summer_reads&utm_campaign=summer_reads_2020_actives&utm_content=20200726&utm_term=all-actives.
89. Sarah Newey, "UK Unveils New 'Global Pandemic Radar' as World Takes Steps to Address Vaccine Inequality," *Telegraph*, May 21, 2021, https://www.telegraph.co.uk/global-health/science-and-disease/uk-unveils-new-global-pandemic-radar-track-covid-variants-spot/.
90. Jennifer Rigby, "WHO and Germany Set Up Global Hub in Bid to Better Fight Next Pandemic," *Telegraph*, May 5, 2021, https://www.telegraph.co.uk/global-health/science-and-disease/germany-set-global-hub-bid-better-fight-next-pandemic/;

WHO, "WHO Hub for Pandemic and Epidemic Intelligence," accessed December 30, 2021, https://www.who.int/initiatives/who-hub-for-pandemic-and-epidemic-intelligence.

91. Veronique Greenwood, "Scientists Are Trying to Spot New Viruses Before They Cause Pandemics," *New York Times*, February 15, 2021, https://www.nytimes.com/2021/02/15/health/scientists-viruses.html?action=click&module=Spotlight&pgtype=Homepage. See also Mina et al., "A Global Immunological Observatory."

92. Carl Zimmer and Noah Weiland, "C.D.C. Announces $200 Million 'Down Payment' to Track Virus Variants," *New York Times*, February 17, 2021, https://www.nytimes.com/2021/02/17/health/coronavirus-variant-sequencing.html?searchResultPosition=1. On the importance of genomic surveillance, see The Rockefeller Foundation, "Accelerating National Genomic Surveillance," March 2021, https://www.rockefellerfoundation.org/report/accelerating-national-genomic-surveillance/.

93. "Francis DeSouza on the Need."

94. Dan Diamond, Joel Achenbach, Chico Harlan, and Lesley Wroughton, "'You've Got to Prepare for the Worst': World Responds to New Variant's Arrival," *Washington Post*, November 27, 2021, https://www.washingtonpost.com/world/covid-variant-fallout-omnicron/2021/11/27/8c6e0548-4f02-11ec-a7b8-9ed28bf23929_story.html.

95. Maureen Miller, "The Next Pandemic Is Already Happening—Targeted Disease Surveillance Can Help Prevent It," *The Conversation*, June 1, 2021, https://theconversation.com/the-next-pandemic-is-already-happening-targeted-disease-surveillance-can-help-prevent-it-160429.

96. GLEWS, "About GLEWS," accessed December 30, 2021, http://www.glews.net/?page_id=5.

97. Julie Flaherty, "A Push to Prevent the Next Pandemic," *Tufts Now*, October 7, 2020, https://now.tufts.edu/articles/push-prevent-next-pandemic.

98. Amos Zeeberg, "Piecing Together the Next Pandemic," *New York Times*, February 16, 2021, https://www.nytimes.com/2021/02/16/health/coronavirus-pandemic-cambodia-manning.html?searchResultPosition=1.

99. For an example of social media monitoring, see Lopreite et al., "Early Warnings of COVID-19?" On modeling and AI, see Carly S. Cox et al., "Summary Report of the National Summit on the Science and Technology of Epidemiological Modeling and Prediction," Institute for Defense Analyses, December 2020, https://www.cdc.gov/nchs/data/misc/STPI-Epi-Modeling-Summit-Report-01-14-2021.pdf; and NSCAI, "The Role of AI Technology in Pandemic Response and Preparedness: Recommended Investments and Initiatives," White Paper Series on Pandemic Response and Preparedness, June 2020.

100. I am grateful to Patrick Walsh for his discussion with me on this point.

101. Richard Galpin, "Big Data 'Can Stop Malaria Outbreaks Before They Start,'" *BBC News*, June 10, 2019, https://www.bbc.com/news/health-48581317.

102. Trinity Challenge, "To Ensure We Are Better Prepared Against Health Emergencies," accessed December 30, 2021, https://thetrinitychallenge.org/. See also Sally Davies, Audi, and Cuddihy, "Leveraging Data and New Digital Tools."

103. Rachael Levy, Dan Frosch, and Sadie Gurman, "Capitol Riot Warnings Weren't Acted On as System Failed," *Wall Street Journal Online*, February 8, 2021, https://www.wsj.com/articles/capitol-riot-warnings-werent-acted-on-as-system-failed-11612787596.

104. Vogel, "Intelligent Assessment," 43–44. Clinton has talked in interviews about the influence books such as *The Hot Zone*, by the same author as *The Cobra Event*, had on his thinking about biological warfare and pandemics; see, for example, his interview on *Late Night with Seth Meyers*, June 24, 2021, https://www.youtube.com/watch?v=zxjxPCMBdw4.

105. Matthew Mosk, "George W. Bush in 2005: 'If We Wait for a Pandemic to Appear, It Will Be Too Late to Prepare,'" *ABC News* April 5, 2020, https://abcnews.go.com/amp/Politics/george-bush-2005-wait-pandemic-late-prepare/story?id=69979013. See also Karl Rove, "Clinton and Bush Prepared for Pandemics," *Wall Street Journal*, April 8, 2020, https://www.wsj.com/articles/clinton-and-bush-prepared-for-pandemics-11586387379.

106. Wirtz, "COVID-19," 6.

107. Dahl, *Intelligence and Surprise Attack*, 110–27.

108. Jervis, "Why Intelligence and Policymakers Clash," 196.

109. Lankford, Storzieri, and Fitsanakis, "Spies and the Virus," 107.

110. Lankford, Storzieri, and Fitsanakis, 9.

111. Jack Davis, "The Challenge of Opportunity Analysis."

112. Lowenthal, *Intelligence*, 5.

113. Dahl, "Why Won't They Listen?," 84.

114. Lowenthal, "Grant vs. Sherman," 198.

115. Pellerin, "Medical Intelligence Center Monitors Health Threats."

116. Cited in Wesley Wark, "The System Was Not Blinking Red: Intelligence, Early Warning and Risk Assessment in a Pandemic Crisis," Centre for International Governance Innovation, August 24, 2020, https://www.cigionline.org/articles/system-was-not-blinking-red-intelligence-early-warning-and-risk-assessment-pandemic-crisis.

117. Hassan et al., "Hindsight Is 2020?," 397.

118. Peter M. Sandman, "Public Health's Share of the Blame: US COVID-19 Risk Communication Failures," University of Minnesota Center for Infectious Disease Research and Policy, August 24, 2020, https://www.cidrap.umn.edu/news-perspective/2020/08/commentary-public-healths-share-blame-us-covid-19-risk-communication.

119. Bowsher and Sullivan, "Why We Need."

120. Danielle Allen, "Democracy, Autocracy, and the Pandemic," *Foreign Affairs* webinar, June 25, 2020, https://www.foreignaffairs.com/events/2020-06-25/foreign-affairs-julyaugust-2020-issue-launch-democracy-autocracy-and-pandemic. See also Allen, "A More Resilient Union."

121. Freedman, "Scientific Advice."

122. Lawrence Freedman, "Written Evidence Submitted by Sir Lawrence Freedman," September 7, 2020, https://committees.parliament.uk/writtenevidence/11273/pdf/.

123. This section draws upon Dahl, "Warnings Unheeded, Again."

124. Emily Anthes, "The Future of Virus Tracking Can Be Found on This College Campus," *New York Times*, May 17, 2021, https://www.nytimes.com/2021/05/17/health/coronavirus-broad-colorado-mesa-sabeti.html?action=click&module=Well&pgtype=Homepage&section=Health; Susan Landau, "Lessons from Contact-Tracing and Exposure-Notification Apps," *Lawfare* (blog), May 26, 2021, https://www.lawfareblog.com/lessons-contact-tracing-and-exposure-notification-apps.

125. Boudreaux et al., "Data Privacy During Pandemics"; Clark, Chiao, and Amirian, "Why Contact Tracing."

126. Susan Landau, "Contact-Tracing Apps Have Serious Physical, Biological Limitations," *Big Think* (blog), May 24, 2021, https://bigthink.com/coronavirus/contact-tracing-apps-have-serious-physical-biological-limitations.
127. This is the argument in Bernard, Bowsher, and Sullivan, "COVID-19 and the Rise."
128. Jha, "System Failure," 112.
129. See, for example, Access Now, "Recommendations on Privacy and Data Protection in the Fight Against COVID-19," March 2020, https://www.accessnow.org/cms/assets/uploads/2020/03/Access-Now-recommendations-on-Covid-and-data-protection-and-privacy.pdf; Bagchi et al., "Digital Tools for COVID-19."
130. International Commission of Jurists, "Siracusa Principles."
131. Rushton, *Security and Public Health*, 115; Sun, "Applying Siracusa."
132. Bernard et al., "Intelligence and Global Health."
133. Bernard et al., 512. For a useful discussion of these issues, see Jessica Davis, "Surveillance, Intelligence."

# CONCLUSION

## A Wake-Up Call for Humanity

I have argued here that the coronavirus pandemic beginning in 2019 was largely the result of a global failure of intelligence and warning. This failure occurred at many levels, including within the traditional intelligence community, which especially in the United States found itself reporting too little, too late on the outbreak. Even more important were the failures of the medical and public health intelligence, surveillance, and warning systems, which were not prepared to provide the kind of near-real-time data on the spread of the virus that was needed by decision-makers.

This crisis has taught us many important lessons about how we can do better next time, when the experts tell us we likely will face an even more dangerous pandemic. One of those lessons is that long-term strategic warning of a threat is of little value on its own, primarily because decision-makers are typically focused on near-term challenges. Strategic warnings, such as those that come through national intelligence assessments, reports by think tanks, or studies by blue-ribbon commissions, provide value only to the extent that they raise awareness of threats and lead to the development of systems that can produce actionable, tactical intelligence when a threat actually develops. But none of this matters if decision-makers—who may be national leaders or local public health officials—are not trained or experienced enough to be able to understand and be receptive to the warnings they receive.

A second lesson from the global crisis is that in the future the different realms of intelligence—national security, medical, and public health—will need to coordinate much more closely if the world wants to be prepared to anticipate and prevent the next pandemic. This closer coordination will lead to direct benefits, such as improved sharing of information on future outbreaks, but it will also lead to broader and longer-term benefits, as professionals in these different fields learn valuable lessons from each other about how to better think about and anticipate threats. For example, medical and public health professionals can benefit from understanding the intelligence cycle and how important it is to develop a strong relationship between intelligence and policy makers before a threat arises.

The most important lesson from the current crisis, however, is that global threats will arise from literally anywhere in the world, and the increasing interconnectivity of all of us—what is sometimes described as globalization—puts everyone on the planet at greater risk from a wider array of threats than ever before in human history. Although many have predicted that globalization will suffer as a result of the crisis, it seems clear that we cannot turn back the clock on global travel and interconnectedness. The world will continue to be "flat," which means that threats will reach us more easily than they have in the past.[1]

The coronavirus pandemic needs to serve as a wake-up call for all kinds of threats, whether a biological event or not, and the lessons we have learned about intelligence and warning can be useful as we prepare to face those threats. Besides the pandemic, the global threat that may have received the most attention in recent years is climate change. The director of national intelligence has called it "an urgent national security threat";[2] the US National Intelligence Council has warned that it will increase the risks to US national security;[3] and a wide range of experts and blue-ribbon commissions have warned about the implications of climate change for global security.[4] In what the UN secretary general has called a "code red for humanity," the Intergovernmental Panel on Climate Change released a report in August 2021 that warned that human activities have warmed the climate at a rate unprecedented over at least the past two thousand years.[5]

There is no lack of alarming forecasts about other threats facing humanity and their dangerous possibilities. The DNI's 2021 annual worldwide threat assessment, for example, warned of a "diverse array of threats" that include threats from great powers such as China and Russia; illicit drugs, human trafficking, and transnational crime; mass migration and displaced populations; and cyber threats ranging from nation-states stealing citizens' information to authoritarian regimes around the world using digital tools to surveil their citizens.[6] The NIC has described a series of grim scenarios in which the world faces not only climate change and disease, but financial crises, environmental degradation, and disruptive technologies. In response, the NIC warns, "national security will require not only defending against armies and arsenals but also withstanding and adapting to these shared global challenges."[7] The World Economic Forum has warned that widening inequality and social fragmentation may exacerbate the risks from clear and present dangers such as disease, extreme weather, and terrorist attacks.[8]

To this long list of mostly human-caused dangers we can add a number of other kinds of natural disasters that may pose an existential threat to humanity. Such threats could come in the form of an asteroid impact, a coronal mass ejection from the sun that produces an electromagnetic pulse knocking out electrical systems, or any of a number of other kinds of global-scale natural disasters.[9]

These dangers are what intelligence officials and risk analysts call "high impact, low probability" events. Because they are each individually unlikely to occur at any given time—or at least during a leader's time in office—such threats are difficult to comprehend and address. But, as *The Economist* notes, these events "are a fact of life" and we should plan for them.[10]

Historian Niall Ferguson argues that it is no coincidence that the world is facing a multitude of threats and challenges today, ranging from wildfires to disease to social and political unrest. What appears to be happening, Ferguson writes, is that "our technological advances and demographic expansion have created ideal conditions for significant, life-shortening disasters."[11] As Harvard's Margaret Bourdeaux has described it, these new types of threats— pollution, climate change, cyber attacks, and others—are all existential threats that require global cooperation, and all are exacerbated by inequality in our societies in ways that traditional threats are not.[12]

Although other threats are in many ways quite different from the COVID-19 pandemic under consideration here, in some ways all threats require a similar approach if we are to have any hope of addressing them successfully. Similar to the coronavirus, solutions to these other existential threats require a whole-of-nation approach, but even more than that, they need a global approach.[13]

Some have argued that the world's response to COVID-19 provides hope that we will now be able to respond effectively to other threats, such as climate change.[14] The research conducted for this book suggests the prospect for global cooperation is more in doubt than this optimistic assessment would suggest. But we can take lessons for intelligence, warning, and response from the recent pandemic and apply them to our thinking about future threats. Tim Lord argues that the first lesson we should take from the pandemic is the importance of acting quickly; he notes that countries that moved fast fared much better than those that did not.[15] Lord sees another important lesson, similar to an additional point made here: "'Following the science' is not a strategy. For COVID-19, as for climate, the science will only take you so far."[16]

There is good news, though, because, as a number of experts have noted, the coronavirus pandemic was foreseeable and was indeed foreseen. Similarly, most, or perhaps all of the strategic surprises the United States has faced in recent years have been predictable. They have been described as "known unknowns"—using Donald Rumsfeld's terminology—resulting in shocks or surprises that were recognized before they occurred; they were not "black swans," or only predictable in hindsight, nor "bolts from the blue" that could not reasonably be expected to occur.[17] Very likely the next global crisis, whether it is another pandemic, a human-caused disaster, or a natural catastrophe, has been and is today being predicted. The challenge is to learn how to listen to those predictions and use them to spur the development of intelligence- and information-gathering tools that decision-makers use to guide policymaking in the future.

There is other good news as well, because we now know that some of the efforts that provide early warning of disease and various health threats can be put to use in addressing other types of threats, such as from climate change. For one example, experts argue that global efforts to reduce deforestation could be used to reduce future disease outbreaks while also helping to reduce the ecological impact of deforestation. This is because developments such as the reduction of the rainforest in Brazil, encroachment into wild lands in the United States, and urbanization into wilderness areas in China all serve to remove the natural buffers that maintain the separation between wildlife and people, expanding the possibility for pandemics to emerge.[18] Another effort that is useful in its own right, but which will also help reduce the likelihood of future pandemics, is reducing the world wildlife trade, such as through increased financial support for existing organizations and networks that work to enforce wildlife trade regulations.[19] Tom Friedman argues that the world community needs to work to eliminate illegal wildlife trade that feeds into wet markets, writing: "Loose nukes kill. So can caged pangolins."[20]

What does the US intelligence community need to do to combat these threats? First, it must continue to track and warn of not only the immediate threats facing the country but of the dangers beyond the horizon. Only by having the most expansive (and expensive) intelligence community in history will that be possible, and this means continuing to spend a significant portion of the American national treasure on intelligence.

Second, the IC and the intelligence agencies of allied nations need to broaden their focus and put more attention on nontraditional security threats. Intelligence agencies are already concerned about these issues, of course, and the COVID-19 pandemic has sparked discussion among experts about whether traditional agencies should broaden their focus beyond the human- and state-caused threats that have been their bread and butter for as long as they have existed. Some have already begun to make a significant shift. In Britain the director of MI-6 (counterpart to the US CIA) has said that climate change is now a top priority, arguing that global warming is "the foremost international foreign policy agenda item for this country and for the planet."[21] The role for intelligence, he suggests, might include tracking whether nations live up to their commitments on carbon emissions and other measures to combat climate change.

Not all experts agree with this recommendation; some argue that the intelligence community should not spread itself too thin because its comparative advantage lies in collecting and analyzing secret information. This advantage implies that it may not be appropriate for intelligence agencies to significantly broaden their focus to include nontraditional threats.[22] And making a significant shift in the US intelligence community will require a major change in the culture of intelligence agencies. Former CIA deputy director Michael Morell, for example, has said that nuclear war, pandemics, and climate change all are existential threats to the United States, but "of the three things that are the greatest threat to our existence, we really only focus on one in the Intelligence Community."[23] A key lesson of the pandemic, however, has been that not only can national security threats come from unexpected and nontraditional directions, but also the intelligence and warning about those threats can come from nontraditional sources. Intelligence agencies must now be looking in those directions and developing those sources.

Beyond the realm of intelligence, the United States and its allies must also adopt and embrace a broader definition of national security, to include not only disease but other nontraditional threats like climate change. Some experts, such as Linda Bilmes, are skeptical about whether even the impact of a worldwide pandemic will be enough to change the traditional US approach to national security, which in the past has emphasized state-based threats and military responses. She writes: "Although a small virus has overturned life and well-being across America and the rest of the world, it is not powerful enough to fundamentally reshape how America thinks about national security."[24]

The world's shared experience of the COVID-19 pandemic provides strong evidence that we can and must reshape the way we think about national security, and a crucial step is to reshape the way we think about intelligence and warning. Part of the challenge today is to ask: What expertise and capabilities do we need to develop now so that we will not be looking to create them later, when the next crisis has already hit, whether it is an electromagnetic pulse or something else? Of course, we cannot prepare fully for every potential crisis, but we can develop plans today for how we will respond. As a former science advisor to the British government told *The Economist*, "If what happened at the start of 2020 was a coronal mass ejection that had knocked out the entire technology stack, we would probably be saying, 'Goodness, if only we had more electrical engineers.'"[25]

No government and no society can focus on all threats all the time. So how do we decide which of the many threats are worthy of our focus? We decide by using the concepts of intelligence and warning to identify the most significant future threats and then developing more targeted intelligence-collection and analysis tools to anticipate and detect when those threats will actually arise. At the same time, we train and educate leaders and decision-makers at all levels of government and society to better understand and use those tools, and to be ready to listen when warnings come.

It is important to recall another lesson from the study of intelligence: no matter how good intelligence and warning may be, some threats will always make their way through our defenses, whether those defenses are staffed by military personnel or public health and medical professionals. As renowned intelligence scholar Richard Betts has written, at some point surprise will inevitably succeed despite warning.[26] Betts argues that this suggests the best defense is one that assumes the existence of surprise, and this same advice is often heard from emergency managers and disaster experts. Lucy Jones, for example, argues about earthquake warnings: we should not focus too much on trying to predict when a disaster will happen, but instead on how we will respond when it does.[27]

Preparedness, resiliency, and planning for response are beyond the scope of this book. Nevertheless, even if we are able to improve our intelligence and warning systems for global health threats, intelligence and warning will never be enough and not all threats can be prevented. But, even so, intelligence and warning can play a part in preparing for disaster. It is very likely that tomorrow's catastrophes are already on the radar today, so we should be using those warnings to guide us in planning so that our society will be more resilient when a threat does arise.

The next worldwide threat may well arise from climate change or from some other natural disaster; or, as indicated by the Russian invasion of Ukraine (underway as this book is being completed), it might develop out of a more conventional security crisis resulting from rising tensions among the world's great powers. It could even come from an as-yet-unanticipated direction, although the lessons of strategic warning in past crises strongly suggest that tomorrow's threat will be something we have seen before. No matter the specific vector, the story of the COVID-19 pandemic teaches us that future threats are likely to go global very quickly. For that reason, global as well as national intelligence and warning systems will be needed to anticipate, detect, and respond.

## NOTES

1. For example, see Philippe Legrain, "The Coronavirus Is Killing Globalization as We Know It," *Foreign Policy*, March 12, 2020, https://foreignpolicy.com/2020/03/12/coronavirus-killing-globalization-nationalism-protectionism-trump/.
2. Olivia Gazis, "U.S. Intelligence Touts New Emphasis on Climate Change, Calling It an 'Urgent National Security Threat,'" *CBS News*, April 23, 2021, https://www.cbsnews.com/news/climate-change-national-security-threat-us-intelligence/.
3. NIC, "Climate Change and International Responses."
4. See, for example, Oppenheimer, "As the World Burns"; Kate A. Guy, "A Security Threat Assessment of Global Climate Change," National Security, Military, and Intelligence Panel on Climate Change, February 2020, https://climateandsecurity.org/wp-content/uploads/2020/03/a-security-threat-assessment-of-climate-change.pdf; and Atwoli et al., "Call for Emergency Action."

5. Intergovernmental Panel on Climate Change, "Climate Change 2021," 7.
6. Director of National Intelligence, "Annual Threat Assessment."
7. NIC, "Global Trends 2040," 2.
8. World Economic Forum, "The Global Risks Report 2021."
9. A useful survey is: Global Challenges Foundation: "Global Catastrophic Risks 2021: Navigating the Complex Intersections," October 2021, https://globalchallenges .org/wp-content/uploads/2021/09/Global-Catastrophic-Risks-2021-FINAL.pdf.
10. "The Next Catastrophe: Politicians Ignore Far-Out Risks; They Need to Up Their Game," *The Economist*, June 25, 2020, https://www.economist.com/leaders/2020/06 /25/politicians-ignore-far-out-risks-they-need-to-up-their-game?utm_campaign =the-economist-this-week&utm_medium=newsletter&utm_source=salesforce -marketing-cloud&utm_term=2020-06-25&utm_content=main-text-1.
11. Niall Ferguson, "The World's Cascade of Disasters Is Not a Coincidence," *Bloomberg*, July 25, 2021, https://www.bloomberg.com/opinion/articles/2021-07 -25/niall-ferguson-covid-fires-floods-protests-are-pattern-not-coincidence.
12. Tara O'Toole and Margaret Bourdeaux, "Intelligence Failure?: How Divisions Between Intelligence and Public Health Left Us Vulnerable to a Pandemic," https://www.belfercenter.org/event/intelligence-failure-how-divisions-between -intelligence-and-public-health-left-us-vulnerable.
13. Vikram Venkatram and James Giordano, "The COVID Crisis: Implications for United States—and Global—Biosecurity," Strategic Multilayer Assessment Special Topics Paper, April 22, 2020, https://apps.dtic.mil/sti/pdfs/AD1097149.pdf. See also Isaiah Wilson III, "'Hole' of Government: What COVID-19 Reveals about American National Security Planning," *US Army War College*, May 6, 2020, https://ssi.armywarcollege.edu/wp-content/uploads/2020/05/COVID-19-Hole-of -Govt_Wilson_v1.3_post.pdf.
14. Eric Galbraith and Russ Otto, "Coronavirus Response Proves the World Can Act on Climate Change," *The Conversation* (blog), March 19, 2020, https://the conversation.com/coronavirus-response-proves-the-world-can-act-on-climate -change-133999.
15. Tim Lord, "COVID-19 and Climate Change: How to Apply the Lessons of the Pandemic to the Climate Emergency," Tony Blair Institute for Global Change, April 7, 2021, 5, https://institute.global/policy/covid-19-and-climate-change-how-apply -lessons-pandemic-climate-emergency.
16. Lord, 14.
17. Nathan Freier, Robert Hume, and John Schaus, "Memorandum for SECDEF: Restore 'Shock' in Strategic Planning," *US Army War College*, May 5, 2020, https:// ssi.armywarcollege.edu/wp-content/uploads/2020/05/COVID-19-Shocks_Freier _Hume_Schaus_v1.3_post.pdf.
18. Dobson et al., "Ecology and Economics for Pandemic Prevention."
19. Dobson et al., "Ecology and Economics for Pandemic Prevention."
20. Thomas L. Friedman, "One Year Later, We Still Have No Plan to Prevent the Next Pandemic," *New York Times*, March 16, 2021, https://www.nytimes.com/2021 /03/16/opinion/covid-pandemic.html?action=click&module=Opinion&pgtype= Homepage.
21. Tom Newton Dunn, "We Warned Putin What Would Happen If He Invaded Ukraine," *Sunday Times*, April 25, 2021, https://www.thetimes.co.uk/article/mi6s -c-we-warned-putin-what-would-happen-if-he-invaded-ukraine-wkc0m96qn.

22. Joshua Rovner, "Think Small: Why the Intelligence Community Should Do Less About New Threats," *War on the Rocks* (blog), June 16, 2021, https://warontherocks .com/2021/06/think-small-why-the-intelligence-community-should-do-less -about-new-threats/.

23. Michael R. Gordon and Warren P. Strobel, "Coronavirus Pandemic Stands to Force Changes in U.S. Spy Services," *Wall Street Journal*, November 22, 2020, https:// www.wsj.com/articles/coronavirus-pandemic-stands-to-force-changes-in-u-s -spy-services-11606041000.

24. Bilmes, "Rethinking U.S. National Security," 9.

25. "How British Science Came to the Rescue," *The Economist*, February 27, 2021, https://www.economist.com/britain/2021/02/27/how-british-science-came-to -the-rescue.

26. Betts, "Surprise Despite Warning."

27. Lucy Jones, "Catastrophes Like a San Andreas Earthquake Are Inevitable; We Should Plan for Them," *Washington Post*, August 13, 2020, https://www.washington post.com/opinions/2020/08/13/catastrophes-like-san-andreas-earthquake-are -inevitable-we-should-plan-them/?utm_source=twitter&utm_medium=social& utm_campaign=wp_opinions.

# APPENDIX

Timeline of Coronavirus Warning and Response

| Date | Event |
|------|-------|
| **Dec 8, 2019** | First patient in China confirmed to have COVID-19 develops symptoms.[1] |
| **Dec 30** | Wuhan Municipal Health Commission issues its first alert to hospitals about cases of pneumonia of unknown origin.[2] |
| **Dec 30** | Wuhan doctor Li Wenliang writes in an online chat group about a new mystery illness that had infected seven patients at a local hospital. He is silenced by Chinese authorities and later dies of COVID-19.[3] |
| **Dec 30** | HealthMap and ProMED issue alerts about reports of an unusual disease outbreak in Wuhan, the first English-language news reports on the virus.[4] |
| **Dec 31** | WHO office in Beijing reports to the WHO that cases of pneumonia of an unknown cause had been detected in Wuhan.[5] |
| **Dec 31** | More public-health-surveillance systems report on the virus. |
| **Jan 4, 2020** | WHO releases Twitter alert, its first public statement about the outbreak.[6] |
| **Jan 5** | WHO releases first formal alert about a "pneumonia of unknown cause."[7] |
| **Jan 6** | CDC warns Americans to take precautions if traveling to China.[8] |
| **Jan 8** | CDC issues Health Alert Network alert.[9] |
| **Jan 13** | First confirmed case of COVID-19 outside China is confirmed in Thailand.[10] |
| **Jan 14** | WHO releases statement that "there is no clear evidence of human-to-human transmission."[11] |
| **Jan 20** | First US case confirmed by CDC (patient had arrived in Seattle area on January 19).[12] |
| **Jan 23** | First Oval Office briefing to the president that discusses the disease; the briefer downplays the threat.[13] |
| **Jan 29** | Trump announces creation of the President's Coronavirus Task Force.[14] |
| **Jan 30** | WHO declares Public Health Emergency of International Concern.[15] |
| **Jan 31** | Trump suspends entry into United States by foreign nationals who traveled to China, to take effect February 2; the order does not apply to US residents or their family members.[16] |
| **Feb 7** | Trump is interviewed by journalist Bob Woodward; says "This is deadly stuff."[17] |
| **Feb 24** | First documented case of community transmission in United States is detected by Seattle Flu Study.[18] |
| **Feb 25** | NCMI raises pandemic warning from WATCHCON 2 to WATCHCON 1.[19] |
| **Feb 27** | Intelligence briefing to Joint Chiefs of Staff states the virus will "likely" become pandemic within next 30 days.[20] |
| **Feb 29** | First death in United States related to the virus is reported in Washington State.[21] (Later it was determined that several others had died earlier.[22]) |
| **March 11** | WHO declares the virus is a pandemic.[23] |
| **March 16** | White House announces guidelines restricting large gatherings.[24] |

1. Singh et al., "How an Outbreak Became a Pandemic," 2111. Earlier reports had indicated the first patient developed symptoms on December 1, but subsequent evidence suggests he had been infected at a later date. Note that later studies suggest the first (or index) case may have been identified on December 10; see Pekar, "Sars-Cov-2 Emergence."

2. Singh et al., 2112.

3. Gerry Shih, "Chinese Doctor Who Tried to Raise Alarm on Coronavirus in Wuhan Dies on 'Front Line' of Medical Fight," *Washington Post*, February 6, 2020, https://www.washingtonpost.com/world/asia_pacific /chinese-doctor-who-tried-to-raise-alarm-on-coronavirus-in-wuhan-dies-from-disease/2020/02/06/8bf 305a2-48f9-11ea-8a1f-de1597be6cbc_story.html.

4. Associated Press, "China Investigates Respiratory Illness Outbreak Sickening 27," December 30, 2019, https:// apnews.com/article/00c78d1974410d96fe031f67edbd86ec; ProMED, "Undiagnosed Pneumonia—China (Hubei): Request for Information," *ProMED Mail Post* (blog), December 30, 2019, https://promedmail.org /promed-post/?id=6864153; Adrian Cho, "Artificial Intelligence Systems Aim to Sniff Out Signs of COVID-19 Outbreaks," *Science*, May 12, 2020, https://www.science.org/content/article/artificial-intelligence-systems -aim-sniff-out-signs-covid-19-outbreaks.

5. WHO, "COVID-19—China," January 5, 2020, https://www.who.int/csr/don/05-january-2020-pneumonia-of -unkown-cause-china/en/.

6. @WHO, "China Has Reported to WHO a Cluster of Pneumonia Cases," January 4, 2020, https://twitter.com /who/status/1213523866703814656?lang=en.

7. WHO, "COVID-19—China," January 5, 2020, https://www.who.int/csr/don/05-january-2020-pneumonia-of -unkown-cause-china/en/.

8. Susan V. Lawrence, "COVID-19 and China: A Chronology of Events (December 2019–January 2020)," Congressional Research Service, May 13, 2020, 23, https://crsreports.congress.gov/product/pdf/r/r46354.

9. CDC, "Outbreak of Pneumonia of Unknown Etiology (PUE) in Wuhan, China," January 8, 2020, https:// emergency.cdc.gov/han/han00424.asp.

10. WHO, "WHO Statement on Novel Coronavirus in Thailand," January 13, 2020, https://www.who.int/news /item/13-01-2020-who-statement-on-novel-coronavirus-in-thailand.

11. @WHO, "Preliminary Investigations Conducted by the Chinese Authorities," January 14, 2020, https://twitter .com/WHO/status/1217043229427761152.

12. Holshue et al., "First Case of 2019."

13. Julian E. Barnes and Adam Goldman, "For Spy Agencies, Briefing Trump Is a Test of Holding His Attention," *New York Times*, May 28, 2020, https://www.nytimes.com/2020/05/21/us/politics/presidents-daily-brief-trump .html.

14. Lawrence, "COVID-19 and China," 42.

15. Singh et al., "How an Outbreak Became a Pandemic," 2113.

16. Lawrence, "COVID-19 and China," 42.

17. Robert Costa and Philip Rucker, "Woodward Book: Trump Says He Knew Coronavirus was 'Deadly' and Worse than the Flu While Intentionally Misleading Americans," *Washington Post*, September 9, 2020, https:// www.washingtonpost.com/politics/bob-woodward-rage-book-trump/2020/09/09/0368fe3c-efd2-11ea-b4bc -3a2098fc73d4_story.html.

18. Chu et al., "Early Detection."

19. Deb Reichmann, "Medical Intelligence Sleuths Tracked, Warned of New Virus," Associated Press, April 15, 2020, https://apnews.com/article/da45eec432d6ff4cc9e0825531e454a6.

20. Jenni Fink and Naveed Jamali, "Defense Department Expects Coronavirus Will 'Likely' Become Global Pandemic in 30 Days, as Trump Strikes Serious Tone," *Newsweek*, March 1, 2020, https://www.newsweek .com/coronavirus-department-defense-pandemic-30-days-1489876.

21. Dakin Andone, Jamie Gumbrecht, and Michael Nedelman, "First Death from Coronavirus Confirmed in Washington State," CNN, February 29, 2020, https://www.cnn.com/2020/02/29/health/us-coronavirus -saturday/index.html.

22. Benjamin Mueller, "When Was the First U.S. Covid Death?: C.D.C. Investigates 4 Early Cases," *New York Times*, September 9, 2021, https://www.nytimes.com/2021/09/09/health/first-covid-deaths.html?search ResultPosition=1.

23. WHO, "WHO Director-General's Opening Remarks at the Media Briefing on COVID-19," March 11, 2020, https://www.who.int/director-general/speeches/detail/who-director-general-s-opening-remarks-at-the -media-briefing-on-covid-19-11-march-2020.

24. Katie Rogers and Emily Cochrane, "Trump Urges Limits Amid Pandemic, But Stops Short of National Mandates," *New York Times*, March 16, 2020, https://www.nytimes.com/2020/03/16/us/politics/trump -coronavirus-guidelines.html.

# BIBLIOGRAPHY

Abraham, Thomas. "The Chronicle of a Disease Foretold: Pandemic H1N1 and the Construction of a Global Health Security Threat." *Political Studies* 59, no. 4 (November 7, 2011): 797–812. https://doi.org/10.1111/j.1467-9248.2011.00925.x.

Alagoz, Oguzhan, Ajay Sethi, Brian Patterson, Matthew Churpek, and Nasia Safdar. "Impact of Timing of and Adherence to Social Distancing Measures on COVID-19 Burden in the US: A Simulation Modeling Approach." *MedRxiv*, January 1, 2020. https://doi.org/10.1101/2020.06.07.20124859.

Allen, Danielle. "A More Resilient Union: How Federalism Can Protect Democracy from Pandemics." *Foreign Affairs* 99, no 4 (July-August 2020): 33–38.

Atwoli, Lukoye, Abdullah H. Baqui, Thomas Benfield, Raffaella Bosurgi, Fiona Godlee, Stephen Hancocks, Richard Horton, et al. "Call for Emergency Action to Limit Global Temperature Increases, Restore Biodiversity, and Protect Health." *Lancet* 398, no. 10304 (September 11, 2021): 939–41. https://doi.org/10.1016/S0140-6736(21)01915-2.

Auditor General of Canada. "COVID-19 Pandemic Report 8: Pandemic, Surveillance, and Border Control Measures." Independent Auditor's Report, March 2021. https://www.oag-bvg.gc.ca/internet/English/parl_oag_202103_03_e_43785.html.

Australian Department of Defence. "Submission to the Senate Foreign Affairs, Defence and Trade References Committee: Health Preparation Arrangements for ADF Overseas Deployments." Canberra, Australia: Department of Defence, January 13, 2004. https://www.aph.gov.au/~/media/wopapub/senate/committee/fadt_ctte/completed_inquiries/2002_04/defhealth/submissions/sub9_pdf.ashx.

Bagchi, Koustubh "K. J.," Christine Bannan, Sharon Bradford Franklin, Heather Hurlburt, Lauren Sarkesian, Ross Schulman, and Joshua Stager. "Digital Tools for COVID-19 Contact Tracing: Identifying and Mitigating the Equity, Privacy, and Civil Liberties Concerns." White paper. Edmond J. Safra Center for Ethics, July 2, 2020. https://ethics.harvard.edu/digital-tools-for-contact-tracing.

Balcan, Duygu, Bruno Gonçalves, Hao Hu, José J. Ramasco, Vittoria Colizza, and Alessandro Vespignani. "Modeling the Spatial Spread of Infectious Diseases: The Global Epidemic and Mobility Computational Model." *Journal of Computational Science* 1, no. 3 (August 1, 2010): 132–45. https://doi.org/10.1016/j.jocs.2010.07.002.

Baringer, Laura, and Steve Heitkamp. "Securitizing Global Health: A View from Maternal Health." *Global Health Governance* 4, no. 2 (Spring 2011): 1–21. http://blogs.shu.edu/ghg/files/2011/11/Baringer-and-Heitkamp_Securitizing-Global-Health-A-View-from-Maternal-Health_Spring-2011.pdf.

Bar-Joseph, Uri, and Jack S. Levy. "Conscious Action and Intelligence Failure." *Political Science Quarterly* 124, no. 3 (2009): 461–88.

Bar-Joseph, Uri, and Rose McDermott. *Intelligence Success and Failure: The Human Factor*. New York: Oxford University Press, 2017.

Bates, Mary. "Tracking Disease: Digital Epidemiology Offers New Promise in Predicting Outbreaks." *IEEE Pulse* 8, no. 1 (February 2017): 18–22. https://doi.org/10.1109/MPUL.2016.2627238.

Berman, Emily. "The Roles of the State and Federal Governments in a Pandemic." *Journal of National Security Law & Policy* 11, no. 1 (October 2020): 61–82. https://jnslp.com/2020/10/19/the-roles-of-the-state-and-federal-governments-in-a-pandemic/.

Bernard, Kenneth W. "Health and National Security: A Contemporary Collision of Cultures." *Biosecurity and Bioterrorism: Biodefense Strategy, Practice, and Science* 11, no. 2 (June 1, 2013): 157–62. https://doi.org/10.1089/bsp.2013.8522.

Bernard, Rose, G. Bowsher, C. Milner, P. Boyle, P. Patel, and R. Sullivan. "Intelligence and Global Health: Assessing the Role of Open Source and Social Media Intelligence Analysis in Infectious Disease Outbreaks." *Journal of Public Health* 26 (2018): 509–14.

Bernard, Rose, Gemma Bowsher, and Richard Sullivan. "COVID-19 and the Rise of Participatory SIGINT: An Examination of the Rise in Government Surveillance through Mobile Applications." *American Journal of Public Health* 110, no. 12 (December 1, 2020): 1780–85. https://doi.org/10.2105/AJPH.2020.305912.

Bernard, Rose, and Richard Sullivan. "The Use of HUMINT in Epidemics: A Practical Assessment." *Intelligence and National Security* 35, no. 4 (June 6, 2020): 493–501. https://doi.org/10.1080/02684527.2020.1750137.

Betts, Richard K. "Analysis, War, and Decision: Why Intelligence Failures Are Inevitable." *World Politics* 31, no. 1 (October 1978): 61–89.

———. "Surprise Despite Warning: Why Sudden Attacks Succeed." *Political Science Quarterly* 95, no. 4 (1980): 551–72. https://doi.org/10.2307/2150604.

Bilmes, Linda J. "Rethinking U.S. National Security after COVID19." *Peace Economics, Peace Science and Public Policy* 26, no. 3 (2020): 1–11. https://doi.org/10.1515/peps-2020-0055.

Bipartisan Policy Center. "Public Health Forward: Modernizing the U.S. Public Health System." December 2021. https://bipartisanpolicy.org/download/?file=/wp-content/uploads/2021/12/BPC_Public-Health-Forward_R01_WEB.pdf.

Bogoch, Isaac I., Oliver J. Brady, Moritz U. G. Kraemer, Matthew German, Marisa I. Creatore, Manisha A. Kulkarni, John S. Brownstein, et al. "Anticipating the International Spread of Zika Virus from Brazil." *Lancet* 387, no. 10016 (January 23, 2016): 335–36. https://doi.org/10.1016/S0140-6736(16)00080-5.

Bonventre, Eugene V., James B. Peake, and Elizabeth Morehouse. "From Conflict to Pandemics: Three Papers from the CSIS Global Health and Security Working Group." Center for Strategic and International Studies, May 13, 2010. https://www.csis.org/analysis/conflict-pandemics.

Boudreaux, Benjamin, Matthew A. DeNardo, Sarah W. Denton, Ricardo Sanchez, Katie Feistel, and Hardika Dayalani. *Data Privacy During Pandemics: A Scorecard Approach for Evaluating the Privacy Implications of COVID-19 Mobile Phone Surveillance Programs*. Santa Monica, CA: RAND Corporation, 2020. https://doi.org/10.7249/RRA365-1.

Bowsher, Gemma, Rose Bernard, and Richard Sullivan. "A Health Intelligence Framework for Pandemic Response: Lessons from the UK Experience of COVID-19."

*Health Security* 18, no. 6 (September 24, 2020): 435–43. https://doi.org/10.1089/hs .2020.0108.

Bowsher, G., C. Milner, and R. Sullivan. "Medical Intelligence, Security and Global Health: The Foundations of a New Health Agenda." *Journal of the Royal Society of Medicine* 109, no. 7 (2016): 269–73.

Bowsher, Gemma, and Richard Sullivan. "Why We Need an Intelligence-Led Approach to Pandemics: Supporting Science and Public Health during COVID-19 and Beyond." *Journal of the Royal Society of Medicine* 114, no. 1 (September 2, 2020): 12–14. https://doi.org/10.1177/0141076820947052.

Braden, Christopher R., Scott F. Dowell, Daniel B. Jernigan, and James M. Hughes. "Progress in Global Surveillance and Response Capacity 10 Years after Severe Acute Respiratory Syndrome." *Emerging Infectious Diseases* 19, no. 6 (June 2013): 864–69. https://doi.org/10.3201/eid1906.130192.

Brilliant, Larry, Lisa Danzig, Karen Oppenheimer, Agastya Mondal, Rick Bright, and W. Ian Lipkin. "The Forever Virus: A Strategy for the Long Fight against COVID-19." *Foreign Affairs* 100, no. 4 (August 2021): 76–91.

Brower, Jennifer, and Peter Chalk. *The Global Threat of New and Reemerging Infectious Diseases: Reconciling U.S. National Security and Public Health Policy.* Santa Monica, CA: RAND, 2003. https://doi.org/10.7249/MR1602.

Brownstein, John S., Clark C. Freifeld, and Lawrence C. Madoff. "Digital Disease Detection—Harnessing the Web for Public Health Surveillance." *New England Journal of Medicine* 360, no. 21 (May 21, 2009): 2153–57. https://doi.org/10.1056 /NEJMp0900702.

Burans, James, Jennifer S. Goodrich, Robert L. Bull, and Nicholas H. Bergman. "The National Bioforensic Analysis Center." In *Microbial Forensics*, 3rd. ed., edited by Bruce Budowle, Steven Schutzer, and Stephen Morse, 457–61. Cambridge, MA: Academic Press, 2020. https://doi.org/10.1016/B978-0-12-815379-6.00030-1.

Burwell, Sylvia Mathews, Frances Fragos Townsend, Thomas J. Bollyky, and Stewart M. Patrick. "Improving Pandemic Preparedness: Lessons from COVID-19." Independent Task Force Report. New York: Council on Foreign Relations, 2020. https://www.cfr.org/report/pandemic-preparedness-lessons-COVID-19/pdf/TFR _Pandemic_Preparedness.pdf.

Buzan, Barry, Ole Waever, and Jaap de Wilde. *Security: A New Framework for Analysis.* Boulder, CO: Lynne Rienner, 1998.

Calain, Philippe. "From the Field Side of the Binoculars: A Different View on Global Public Health Surveillance." *Health Policy and Planning* 22, no. 1 (January 1, 2007): 13–20. https://doi.org/10.1093/heapol/czl035.

Carey, Warren F., and Myles Maxfield. "Intelligence Implications of Disease." *Studies in Intelligence* 16, no. 1 (Spring 1972): 71–78.

Carney, Timothy Jay, and David Jay Weber. "Public Health Intelligence: Learning from the Ebola Crisis." *American Journal of Public Health* 105, no. 9 (2015): 1740–44.

Carrion, Malwina, and Lawrence C. Madoff. "ProMED-Mail: 22 Years of Digital Surveillance of Emerging Infectious Diseases." *International Health* 9, no. 3 (May 1, 2017): 177–83. https://doi.org/10.1093/inthealth/ihx014.

Cecchine, Gary, and Melinda Moore. "Infectious Disease and National Security: Strategic Information Needs." Technical Report. Santa Monica, CA: RAND, 2006.

Charatan, F. "Eight Die in Outbreak of Virus Spread from Birds." *BMJ (Clinical Research Ed.)* 319, no. 7215 (October 9, 1999): 941. https://doi.org/10.1136/bmj.319.7215.941a.

Chretien, Jean-Paul. "Predictive Surveillance: An Outcome of Applied Interdisciplinary Translational Research in Public Health Surveillance." In *Transforming Public Health Surveillance: Proactive Measures for Prevention, Detection, and Respone,* edited by Scott J. N. McNabb et al., 374–82. Amman, Jordan: Elsevier, 2016.

Chretien, Jean-Paul, Howard S. Burkom, Endang R. Sedyaningsih, Ria P. Larasati, Andres G. Lescano, Carmen C. Mundaca, David L. Blazes, et al. "Syndromic Surveillance: Adapting Innovations to Developing Settings." *PLoS Medicine* 5, no. 3 (March 25, 2008): 0367–72. https://doi.org/10.1371/journal.pmed.0050072.

Christaki, Eirini. "New Technologies in Predicting, Preventing and Controlling Emerging Infectious Diseases." *Virulence* 6, no. 6 (August 18, 2015): 558–65. https://doi.org/10.1080/21505594.2015.1040975.

Chu, Helen Y., Janet A. Englund, Lea M. Starita, Michael Famulare, Elisabeth Brandstetter, Deborah A. Nickerson, Mark J. Rieder, et al. "Early Detection of COVID-19 through a Citywide Pandemic Surveillance Platform." *New England Journal of Medicine* 383, no. 2 (May 1, 2020): 185–87. https://doi.org/10.1056/NEJMc2008646.

CIA (Central Intelligence Agency). "SARS: Lessons from the First Epidemic of the 21st Century." Assessment prepared by Office of Transnational Issues, September 29, 2003. https://www.hsdl.org/?view&did=481435.

———. "Sub-Saharan Africa: Implications of the AIDS Pandemic." Director of Central Intelligence, 1987. https://www.cia.gov/library/readingroom/docs/DOC_0000579143.pdf.

Clapper, James R. "Worldwide Threat Assessment of the US Intelligence Community." Washington, DC: Senate Armed Services Committee, February 26, 2015. https://www.dni.gov/files/documents/Unclassified_2015_ATA_SFR_-_SASC_FINAL.pdf.

Clark, Eva, Elizabeth Y. Chiao, and E. Susan Amirian. "Why Contact Tracing Efforts Have Failed to Curb Coronavirus Disease 2019 (COVID-19) Transmission in Much of the United States." *Clinical Infectious Diseases* 72, no. 9 (May 1, 2021): e415–19. https://doi.org/10.1093/cid/ciaa1155.

Clark, Robert M. *Geospatial Intelligence: Origins and Evolution.* Washington, DC: Georgetown University Press, 2020.

———. *Intelligence Analysis: A Target-Centric Approach.* Thousand Oaks, CA: CQ, 2020.

Clemente, Jonathan D. "CIA's Medical and Psychological Analysis Center (MPAC) and the Health of Foreign Leaders." *International Journal of Intelligence & CounterIntelligence* 19, no. 3 (2006): 385–423.

———. "In Sickness and In Health." *Bulletin of the Atomic Scientists* 63, no. 2 (March 1, 2007): 38–66. https://doi.org/10.2968/063002010.

———. "Medical Intelligence." *Intelligencer* 20, no. 2 (Fall-Winter 2013): 73–78.

Clowers, A. Nicole. "COVID-19: Key Insights from GAO's Oversight of the Federal Public Health Response." Government Accountability Office, February 24, 2021. https://www.gao.gov/assets/gao-21-396t.pdf.

Coats, Daniel R. "Worldwide Threat Assessment of the US Intelligence Community." Senate Select Committee on Intelligence, January 29, 2019. https://www.dni.gov/files/ODNI/documents/2019-ATA-SFR-SSCI.pdf.

Collier, Nigel, Son Doan, Ai Kawazoe, Reiko Matsuda Goodwin, Mike Conway, Yoshio Tateno, Quoc-Hung Ngo, et al. "BioCaster: Detecting Public Health Rumors with a Web-Based Text Mining System." *Bioinformatics (Oxford, England)* 24, no. 24 (December 15, 2008): 2940–41. https://doi.org/10.1093/bioinformatics/btn534.

Conkle, Richard D. "Intelligence Support to Humanitarian Assistance/Disaster Relief Operations." *American Intelligence Journal* 32, no. 2 (2015): 102–6.

Cox, James. "Defence Intelligence and COVID-19." In *Stress Tested: The COVID-19 Pandemic and Canadian National Security*, edited by Leah West, Thomas Juneau, and Amarnath Amarasingam, 161–76. Calgary, Alberta: University of Calgary Press, 2021.

Craven, Matt, et al. "Not the Last Pandemic: Investing Now to Reimaging Public-Health Systems." Atlanta: McKinsey & Company, July 2020. https://www.mckinsey.com /industries/public-and-social-sector/our-insights/not-the-last-pandemic-investing -now-to-reimagine-public-health-systems#

Dahl, Erik J. "Finding Bin Laden: Lessons for a New American Way of Intelligence." *Political Science Quarterly* 129, no. 2 (2014): 179–210.

———. *Intelligence and Surprise Attack: Failure and Success from Pearl Harbor to 9/11 and Beyond*. Washington, DC: Georgetown University Press, 2013.

———. "Local Approaches to Counterterrorism: The New York Police Department Model." *Journal of Policing, Intelligence and Counter Terrorism* 9, no. 2 (July 3, 2014): 81–97. https://doi.org/10.1080/18335330.2014.940815.

———. "The Localization of Intelligence: A New Direction for American Federalism." *International Journal of Intelligence and CounterIntelligence* 34, no. 1 (January 2, 2021): 151–78. https://doi.org/10.1080/08850607.2020.1716563.

———. "Warnings Unheeded, Again: What the Intelligence Lessons of 9/11 Tell Us about the Coronavirus Today." *Homeland Security Affairs* 16 (December 2020): 1–12. https://www.hsaj.org/articles/16304.

———. "Why Won't They Listen?: Comparing Receptivity toward Intelligence at Pearl Harbor and Midway." *Intelligence and National Security* 28, no. 1 (February 1, 2013): 68–90. https://doi.org/10.1080/02684527.2012.749061.

Dai, Yaoyao, and Jianming Wang. "Identifying the Outbreak Signal of COVID-19 before the Response of the Traditional Disease Monitoring System." *PLoS Neglected Tropical Diseases* 14, no. 10 (October 1, 2020): 1–9. https://doi.org/10.1371/journal.pntd .0008758.

Dalglish, Sarah L. "COVID-19 Gives the Lie to Global Health Expertise." *Lancet* 395, no. 10231 (April 11, 2020): 1189. https://doi.org/10.1016/S0140-6736(20)30739-X.

David, Pierre-Marie, and Nicolas Le Dévédec. "Preparedness for the Next Epidemic: Health and Political Issues of an Emerging Paradigm." *Critical Public Health* 29, no. 3 (May 27, 2019): 363–69. https://doi.org/10.1080/09581596.2018.1447646.

Davies, Benjamin, Kaitlin Rainwater Lovett, Brittany Card, and David Polatty. "Urban Outbreak 2019 Pandemic Response: Select Research and Game Findings." Newport, RI: Naval War College, 2020. https://digital-commons.usnwc.edu /civmilresponse-program-sims-uo-2019/2/?utm_source=digital-commons.usnwc .edu%2Fcivmilresponse-program-sims-uo-2019%2F2&utm_medium=PDF&utm _campaign=PDFCoverPages.

Davies, Sally C., Hala Audi, and Mitch Cuddihy. "Leveraging Data and New Digital Tools to Prepare for the Next Pandemic." *Lancet* 397, no. 10282 (April 10, 2021): 1349–50. https://doi.org/10.1016/S0140-6736(21)00680-2.

Davies, Sara E. "Healthy Populations, Political Stability, and Regime Type: Southeast Asia as a Case Study." *Review of International Studies* 40, no. 5 (2014): 859–76.

Davies, Sara E., and Jeremy R. Youde, eds. *The Politics of Surveillance and Response to Disease Outbreaks: The New Frontier for States and Non-State Actors*. Farnham, UK: Ashgate, 2015.

Davis, Jack. "The Challenge of Opportunity Analysis: An Intelligence Monograph." Washington, DC: Center for the Study of Intelligence, July 1992.

Davis, Jessica. "Surveillance, Intelligence and Ethics in a COVID-19 World." In *National Security Intelligence and Ethics*, edited by Seumas Miller, Mitt Regan, and Patrick F. Walsh, 156–66. London: Routledge, 2022.

Dehner, George. "WHO Knows Best?: National and International Responses to Pandemic Threats and the 'Lessons' of 1976." *Journal of the History of Medicine and Allied Sciences* 65, no. 4 (October 2010): 478–513. https://doi.org/10.1093/jhmas/jrq002.

DeLaet, Debra L. "Whose Interests Is the Securitization of Health Serving?." In *Routledge Handbook of Global Health Security*. London: Routledge Handbooks Online, 2014. https://www.routledgehandbooks.com/doi/10.4324/9780203078563.ch28.

Deudney, Daniel. "The Case Against Linking Environmental Degradation and National Security." *Millennium* 19, no. 3 (December 1, 1990): 461–76. https://doi.org/10.1177/03058298900190031001.

DeVine, Michael E. "Intelligence Community Support to Pandemic Preparedness and Response." Congressional Research Service, May 6, 2020. https://crsreports.congress.gov/product/pdf/IF/IF11537.

DHS (Department of Homeland Security). "The 2014 Quadrennial Homeland Security Review." Washington, DC: Department of Homeland Security, 2014. https://www.dhs.gov/sites/default/files/publications/2014-qhsr-final-508.pdf.

Dion, M., P. AbdelMalik, and A. Mawudeku. "Big Data and the Global Public Health Intelligence Network (GPHIN)." *Canada Communicable Disease Report Releve Des Maladies Transmissibles Au Canada* 41, no. 9 (September 3, 2015): 209–14. https://doi.org/10.14745/ccdr.v41i09a02.

Director of National Intelligence (DNI). "Annual Threat Assessment of the US Intelligence Community." February 2022. https://www.dni.gov/files/ODNI/documents/assessments/ATA-2022-Unclassified-Report.pdf.

———. "Annual Threat Assessment of the US Intelligence Community." April 9, 2021. https://www.dni.gov/files/ODNI/documents/assessments/ATA-2021-Unclassified-Report.pdf.

———. "Intelligence Community Directive 204: National Intelligence Priorities Framework." January 7, 2021. https://www.dni.gov/files/documents/ICD/ICD_204_National_Intelligence_Priorities_Framework_U_FINAL-SIGNED.pdf.

———. "Updated Assessment on COVID-19 Origins." October 29, 2021. https://www.dni.gov/files/ODNI/documents/assessments/Declassified-Assessment-on-COVID-19-Origins.pdf.

Dobson, Andrew P., Stuart L. Pimm, Lee Hannah, Les Kaufman, Jorge A. Ahumada, Amy W. Ando, Aaron Bernstein, et al. "Ecology and Economics for Pandemic Prevention." *Science* 369, no. 6502 (July 24, 2020): 379. https://doi.org/10.1126/science.abc3189.

Duff, Johnathan H., Anicca Liu, Jorge Saavedra, Jacob N. Batycki, Kendra Morancy, Barbara Stocking, Lawrence O. Gostin, et al. "A Global Public Health Convention for the 21st Century." *Lancet Public Health* 6, no. 6 (June 1, 2021): e428–33. https://doi.org/10.1016/S2468-2667(21)00070-0.

Elbe, Stefan. "Haggling over Viruses: The Downside Risks of Securitizing Infectious Disease." *Health Policy and Planning* 25, no. 6 (November 1, 2010): 476–85. https://doi.org/10.1093/heapol/czq050.

———. "Should Health Professionals Play the Global Health Security Card?." *Lancet* 377 (July 16, 2011): 220–21.

Enemark, Christian. *Biosecurity Dilemmas: Dreaded Diseases, Ethical Responses, and the Health of Nations*. Washington, DC: Georgetown University Press, 2017.

———. "Is Pandemic Flu a Security Threat?." *Survival* 51, no. 1 (March 1, 2009): 191–214. https://doi.org/10.1080/00396330902749798.

Fairchild, Amy L., Ronald Bayer, and James Colgrove. *Searching Eyes: Privacy, the State, and Disease Surveillance in America*. Berkeley, CA: University of California Press, 2007.

Faure, Nicolaas Mattheus, Chloe Hupin, Xavier Deparis, and Marc Tanti. "How Did the Medical Intelligence Unit Handle the Influenza Pandemic in the French Armed Forces in 2009?." Third International Symposium ISKO, the Maghreb, 2013. https://ieeexplore.ieee.org/document/6728114.

Fearnley, Lyle. "Redesigning Syndromic Surveillance for Biosecurity." In *Biosecurity Interventions*, edited by Andrew Lakoff and Stephen Collier, 61–88. New York: Columbia University Press, 2008. https://doi.org/10.7312/lako14606-003.

Feldbaum, Harley, Preeti Patel, Egbert Sondorp, and Kelley Lee. "Global Health and National Security: The Need for Critical Engagement." *Medicine, Conflict and Survival* 22, no. 3 (July 1, 2006): 192–98. https://doi.org/10.1080/13623690600772501.

Fellner, Chris. "Zika in America: The Year in Review." *P & T: A Peer-Reviewed Journal for Formulary Management* 41, no. 12 (December 2016): 778–91.

FEMA (Federal Emergency Management Agency). "2019 National Threat and Hazard Identification and Risk Assessment (THIRA): Overview and Methodology." July 25, 2019. https://www.hsdl.org/?view&did=827415.

Fergie, Dexter. "Geopolitics Turned Inwards: The Princeton Military Studies Group and the National Security Imagination." *Diplomatic History* 43, no. 4 (2019): 644–70.

Ferguson, Niall. *Doom: The Politics of Catastrophe*. New York: Penguin, 2021.

Fineberg, Harvey V. "Pandemic Preparedness and Response—Lessons from the H1N1 Influenza of 2009." *New England Journal of Medicine* 370 (April 3, 2014): 1335–42. https://doi.org/10.1056/NEJMra1208802.

———. "Report of the Review Committee on the Functioning of the International Health Regulations (2005) in Relation to Pandemic (H1N1) 2009." World Health Organization, May 5, 2011. https://apps.who.int/gb/ebwha/pdf_files/WHA64/A64_10-en.pdf.

———. "Swine Flu of 1976: Lessons from the Past." *Bulletin of the World Health Organization* 87, no. 6 (June 2009). https://www.who.int/bulletin/volumes/87/6/09-040609/en/.

Fischhoff, Baruch. "Communicating Uncertainty: Fulfilling the Duty to Inform." *Issues in Science and Technology* 28, no. 4 (Summer 2012). https://issues.org/fischhoff/#.YJcFHSNJS8k.link.

Fitch, J. Patrick. "National Biodefense Analysis and Countermeasures Center." In *Encyclopedia of Bioterrorism Defense*. Hoboken, NJ: John Wiley & Sons, 2011. https://onlinelibrary.wiley.com/doi/abs/10.1002/0471686786.ebd0174.

Foege, William H., Robert C. Hogan, and Ladene H. Newton. "Surveillance Projects for Selected Diseases." *International Journal of Epidemiology* 5, no. 1 (March 1, 1976): 29–37. https://doi.org/10.1093/ije/5.1.29.

Freedman, Lawrence. "Scientific Advice at a Time of Emergency: SAGE and COVID-19." *Political Quarterly* 91, no. 3 (July 1, 2020): 514–22. https://doi.org/10.1111/1467-923X.12885.

Freifeld, Clark C., Kenneth D. Mandl, Ben Y. Reis, and John S. Brownstein. "HealthMap: Global Infectious Disease Monitoring through Automated Classification and Visualization of Internet Media Reports." *Journal of the American Medical Informatics Association* 15, no. 2 (March 1, 2008): 150–57. https://doi.org/10.1197/jamia.M2544.

French, Martin A. "Woven of War-Time Fabrics: The Globalization of Public Health Surveillance." *Surveillance & Society* 6, no. 2 (February 27, 2009): 101–15. https://doi.org/10.24908/ss.v6i2.3251.

Frieden, Thomas R. "The Future of Public Health." *New England Journal of Medicine* 373, no. 18 (October 28, 2015): 1748–54. https://doi.org/10.1056/NEJMsa1511248.

Frieden, Thomas R., Christopher T. Lee, Aaron F. Bochner, Marine Buissonnière, and Amanda McClelland. "7-1-7: An Organising Principle, Target, and Accountability Metric to Make the World Safer from Pandemics." *Lancet* 398, no. 10300 (August 14, 2021): 638–40. https://doi.org/10.1016/S0140-6736(21)01250-2.

Frommelt, Paul. "Defense Watch: NGA Supports Ebola Crisis." *Earth Imaging Journal*, February 21, 2015. https://eijournal.com/print/column/defense-watch/nga-supports-ebola-crisis.

Fuerth, Leon. "Operationalizing Anticipatory Governance." *Prism* 2, no. 4 (September 2011): 31–46.

Gardy, Jennifer L., and Nicholas J. Loman. "Towards a Genomics-Informed, Real-Time, Global Pathogen Surveillance System." *Nature Reviews Genetics* 19, no. 1 (January 1, 2018): 9–20. https://doi.org/10.1038/nrg.2017.88.

Garrett, Laurie. "Ebola's Lessons: How the WHO Mishandled the Crisis." *Foreign Affairs* 94, no. 5 (October 2015): 80–107.

———. "The Return of Infectious Disease." *Foreign Affairs* 75, no. 1 (February 1996): 66–79.

Garrett-Cherry, Tiana A., Andrew K. Hennenfent, Sasha McGee, and John Davies-Cole. "Enhanced One Health Surveillance during the 58th Presidential Inauguration—District of Columbia, January 2017." *Disaster Medicine and Public Health Preparedness* 14, no. 2 (2020): 201–7. https://doi.org/10.1017/dmp.2019.38.

Gates, Bill. "The Next Epidemic—Lessons from Ebola." *New England Journal of Medicine* 372, no. 15 (March 18, 2015): 1381–84. https://doi.org/10.1056/NEJMp1502918.

Gentry, John A. "Has the ODNI Improved U.S. Intelligence Analysis?." *International Journal of Intelligence and CounterIntelligence* 28, no. 4 (October 2, 2015): 637–61. https://doi.org/10.1080/08850607.2015.1050937.

Gentry, John A., and Joseph S. Gordon. *Strategic Warning Intelligence: History, Challenges, and Prospects*. Washington, DC: Georgetown University Press, 2019.

Global Preparedness Monitoring Board. "A World at Risk: Annual Report on Global Preparedness for Health Emergencies." Geneva, Switzerland, September 2019. https://apps.who.int/gpmb/assets/annual_report/GPMB_annualreport_2019.pdf.

Gore, Al. "Emerging Infections Threaten National and Global Security." Presented at the National Council for International Health, Arlington, VA, June 12, 1996. https://1997-2001.state.gov/global/oes/health/task_force/article.html.

Gostin, Lawrence O. "The Coronavirus Pandemic 1 Year On—What Went Wrong?." *JAMA* 325, no. 12 (March 23, 2021): 1132–33. https://doi.org/10.1001/jama.2021.3207.

Gostin, Lawrence O., Mary C. DeBartolo, and Eric A. Friedman. "The International Health Regulations 10 Years On: The Governing Framework for Global Health

Security." *Lancet* 386, no. 10009 (November 28, 2015): 2222–26. https://doi.org/10 .1016/S0140-6736(15)00948-4.

Gould, Deborah W., David Walker, and Paula W. Yoon. "The Evolution of BioSense: Lessons Learned and Future Directions." *Public Health Reports* 132, no. 1 (July 1, 2017): 7S-11S. https://doi.org/10.1177/0033354917706954.

GPHIN (Global Public Health Intelligence Network). "Independent Review Panel Final Report." May 28, 2021. https://www.canada.ca/content/dam/phac-aspc/documents /corporate/mandate/about-agency/external-advisory-bodies/list/independent -review-global-public-health-intelligence-network/final-report/final-report-en.pdf.

Gradon, Kacper, and Wesley R. Moy. "COVID-19 Response—Lessons from Secret Intelligence Failures." *International Journal of Intelligence, Security, and Public Affairs*, September 30, 2021, 1–19. https://doi.org/10.1080/23800992.2021.1956776.

Gressang, Daniel S., and James J. Wirtz. "Rethinking Warning: Intelligence, Novel Events, and the COVID-19 Pandemic." *International Journal of Intelligence and CounterIntelligence* 35, no. 1 (January 2, 2022): 131–46. https://doi.org/10.1080 /08850607.2021.1913023.

Gronvall, Gigi Kwik. "The Scientific Response to COVID-19 and Lessons for Security." *Survival* 62, no. 3 (May 3, 2020): 77–92. https://doi.org/10.1080/00396338.2020 .1763613.

Groseclose, Samuel L., and David L. Buckeridge. "Public Health Surveillance Systems: Recent Advances in Their Use and Evaluation." *Annual Review of Public Health* 38, no. 1 (March 20, 2017): 57–79. https://doi.org/10.1146/annurev-publhealth-031816 -044348.

Guglielmetti, P., D. Coulombier, G. G. Thinus, F. Van Loock, and S. Schreck. "The Early Warning and Response System for Communicable Diseases in the EU: An Overview from 1999 to 2005." *Eurosurveillance* 11, no. 12 (2006): 7–8. https://doi.org/10 .2807/esm.11.12.00666-en.

Haftendorn, Helga. "The Security Puzzle: Theory-Building and Discipline-Building in International Security." *International Studies Quarterly* 35, no. 1 (1991): 3–17. https://doi.org/10.2307/2600386.

Hagen, Katie S., Ronald D. Fricker, Krista D. Hanni, Susan Barnes, and Kristy Michie. "Assessing the Early Aberration Reporting System's Ability to Locally Detect the 2009 Influenza Pandemic." *Statistics, Politics, and Policy* 2, no. 1 (2011). https://doi .org/10.2202/2151-7509.1018.

Hagopian, Amy. "Why Isn't War Properly Framed and Funded as a Public Health Problem?." *Medicine, Conflict and Survival* 33, no. 2 (2017): 92–100.

Hartley, D. M., N. P. Nelson, R. R. Arthur, P. Barboza, N. Collier, N. Lightfoot, J. P. Linge, et al. "An Overview of Internet Biosurveillance." *Clinical Microbiology and Infection* 19, no. 11 (November 1, 2013): 1006–13. https://doi.org/10.1111/1469 -0691.12273.

Hartley, D. M., N. P. Nelson, R. Walters, R. Arthur, R. Yangarber, L. Madoff, J. P. Linge, et al. "Landscape of International Event-Based Biosurveillance." *Emerging Health Threats Journal* 3 (2010): 1–7. https://doi.org/10.3134/ehtj.10.003.

Hassan, Ines, Mitsuru Mukaigawara, Lois King, Genevie Fernandes, and Devi Sridhar. "Hindsight Is 2020?: Lessons in Global Health Governance One Year into the Pandemic." *Nature Medicine* 27, no. 3 (March 1, 2021): 396–400. https://doi.org/10 .1038/s41591-021-01272-2.

Hatfill, Steven J. "Rapid Validation of Disease Outbreak Intelligence by Small Independent Verification Teams." *Intelligence and National Security* 35, no. 4 (June 6, 2020): 527–38. https://doi.org/10.1080/02684527.2020.1750149.

Henning, Kelly J. "What Is Syndromic Surveillance?." *Morbidity and Mortality Weekly Report* 53 (2004): 7–11.

Heymann, David L., Lincoln Chen, Keizo Takemi, David P. Fidler, Jordan W. Tappero, Mathew J. Thomas, Thomas A. Kenyon, et al. "Global Health Security: The Wider Lessons from the West African Ebola Virus Disease Epidemic." *Lancet* 385, no. 9980 (May 9, 2015): 1884–901. https://doi.org/10.1016/S0140-6736(15)60858-3.

Heymann, David L., and Edmund Howard. "Keeping Our World Safe by Integrating Public Health Surveillance and Health Security." In *Transforming Public Health Surveillance: Proactive Measures for Prevention, Detection, and Response*, edited by Scott J. N. McNabb et al., 126–49. Amman, Jordan: Elsevier, 2016.

Heymann, David L., and Guenael Rodier. "Global Surveillance, National Surveillance, and SARS." *Emerging Infectious Diseases* 10, no. 2 (February 2004): 173–75.

Hodge, James, and Kim Weidenaar. "Public Health Emergencies as Threats to National Security." *Journal of National Security Law & Policy* 9, no. 1 (September 2016): 81–94.

Hoffman, Steven J., and Sarah L. Silverberg. "Delays in Global Disease Outbreak Responses: Lessons from H1N1, Ebola, and Zika." *American Journal of Public Health* 108, no. 3 (March 2018): 329–33.

Holmes, Edward C., Stephen A. Goldstein, Angela L. Rasmussen, David L. Robertson, Alexander Crits-Christoph, Joel O. Wertheim, Simon J. Anthony, et al. "The Origins of SARS-CoV-2: A Critical Review." *Cell* 184, no. 19 (September 16, 2021): 4848–56. https://doi.org/10.1016/j.cell.2021.08.017.

Holshue, Michelle L., Chas DeBolt, Scott Lindquist, Kathy H. Lofy, John Wiesman, Hollianne Bruce, Christopher Spitters, et al. "First Case of 2019 Novel Coronavirus in the United States." *New England Journal of Medicine* 382, no. 10 (January 31, 2020): 929–36. https://doi.org/10.1056/NEJMoa2001191.

Huang, Yanzhong. "Pandemics and Security." In *Routledge Handbook of Global Health Security*. London: Routledge Handbooks Online, 2014. https://www.routledgehandbooks.com/doi/10.4324/9780203078563.ch7.

Huff, Andrew, Toph Allen, Karissa Whiting, Nathan Breit, and Brock Arnold. "FLIRT-ing with Zika: A Web Application to Predict the Movement of Infected Travelers Validated Against the Current Zika Virus Epidemic." *PLoS Currents* 8 (June 10, 2016). https://doi.org/10.1371/currents.outbreaks.711379ace737b7c04c89765342a9a8c9.

Hulnick, Arthur S. "What's Wrong with the Intelligence Cycle." *Intelligence and National Security* 21, no. 6 (December 1, 2006): 959–79. https://doi.org/10.1080/02684520601046291.

Hutwagner, Lori, William Thompson, G. Matthew Seeman, and Tracee Treadwell. "The Bioterrorism Preparedness and Response Early Aberration Reporting System (EARS)." *Journal of Urban Health* 80, no. 2 (June 2003): i89–96. https://doi.org/10.1007/pl00022319.

Ibrahim, Nahla Khamis. "Epidemiologic Surveillance for Controlling COVID-19 Pandemic: Types, Challenges and Implications." *Journal of Infection and Public Health*, August 21, 2020. https://doi.org/10.1016/j.jiph.2020.07.019.

Ilesanmi, Olayinka Stephen, Olufunmilayo Fawole, Patrick Nguku, Abisola Oladimeji, and Okoro Nwenyi. "Evaluation of Ebola Virus Disease Surveillance System in

Tonkolili District, Sierra Leone." *Pan African Medical Journal* 32, no. 1 (January 21, 2019). https://doi.org/10.11604/pamj.supp.2019.32.1.14434.

IMNRC (Institute of Medicine and National Research Council). *Globalization, Biosecurity, and the Future of the Life Sciences.* Washington, DC: National Academies Press, 2006. https://doi.org/10.17226/11567.

Institute of Medicine. *Learning from SARS: Preparing for the Next Disease Outbreak, Workshop Summary.* Washington, DC: National Academies Press, 2004. https://doi.org/10.17226/10915.

——. *Microbial Threats to Health: Emergence, Detection, and Response.* Washington, DC: National Academies Press, 2003. https://doi.org/10.17226/10636.

——. "Perspectives on the Department of Defense Global Emerging Infections Surveillance and Response System: A Program Review." Washington, DC: National Academies Press, 2001. https://www.nap.edu/download/10203.

Intergovernmental Panel on Climate Change. "Climate Change 2021: The Physical Science Basis Summary for Policymakers." Report, August 7, 2021. https://www.ipcc.ch/report/ar6/wg1/downloads/report/IPCC_AR6_WGI_SPM.pdf.

International Commission of Jurists. "Siracusa Principles on the Limitation and Derogation Provisions in the International Covenant on Civil and Political Rights." New York, 1984. https://www.icj.org/siracusa-principles-on-the-limitation-and-derogation-provisions-in-the-international-covenant-on-civil-and-political-rights/.

IPPPR (Independent Panel for Pandemic Preparedness and Response). "COVID-19: Make It the Last Pandemic." Report, May 2021. https://theindependentpanel.org/mainreport/.

Jarcho, Saul. "Historical Perspectives of Medical Intelligence." *Bulletin of the New York Academy of Medicine* 67, no. 5 (October 1991): 501–6.

Jervis, Robert. "Why Intelligence and Policymakers Clash." *Political Science Quarterly* 125, no. 2 (2010): 185–204.

Jha, Ashish K. "System Failure: America Needs a Global Health Policy for the Pandemic Age." *Foreign Affairs* 100, no. 2 (April 2021): 103–15.

Jian, Shu-Wan, Chiu-Mei Chen, Cheng-Yi Lee, and Ding-Ping Liu. "Real-Time Surveillance of Infectious Diseases: Taiwan's Experience." *Health Security* 15, no. 2 (April 1, 2017): 144–53. https://doi.org/10.1089/hs.2016.0107.

Jin, Jiyong, and Joe Thomas Karackattu. "Infectious Diseases and Securitization: WHO's Dilemma." *Biosecurity and Bioterrorism: Biodefense Strategy, Practice, and Science* 9, no. 2 (May 25, 2011): 181–87. https://doi.org/10.1089/bsp.2010.0045.

Johnson, Loch K. "A Conversation with James R. Clapper, Jr., the Director of National Intelligence in the United States." *Intelligence and National Security* 30, no. 1 (January 2015): 1–25. https://doi.org/10.1080/02684527.2014.972613.

Jorden, Michelle A., Sarah L. Rudman, Elsa Villarino, Stacey Hoferka, and Megan T. Patel. "Evidence for Limited Early Spread of COVID-19 Within the United States, January-February 2020." *Morbidity and Mortality Weekly Report* 69 (2020): 680–84.

Kahana, Ephraim. "Intelligence Against COVID-19: Israeli Case Study." *International Journal of Intelligence and CounterIntelligence* 34, no. 2 (April 3, 2021): 259–66. https://doi.org/10.1080/08850607.2020.1783620.

Kahn, David. "The Intelligence Failure of Pearl Harbor." *Foreign Affairs* 70, no. 5 (Winter 1991–92): 138–52.

Kamradt-Scott, Adam. "WHO's to Blame?: The World Health Organization and the 2014 Ebola Outbreak in West Africa." *Third World Quarterly* 37, no. 3 (March 3, 2016): 401–18. https://doi.org/10.1080/01436597.2015.1112232.

Kamradt-Scott, Adam, and Colin McInnes. "The Securitisation of Pandemic Influenza: Framing, Security and Public Policy." *Global Public Health* 7, no. 2 (December 1, 2012): S95–110. https://doi.org/10.1080/17441692.2012.725752.

Keller, Mikaela, Michael Blench, Herman Tolentino, Clark C. Freifeld, Kenneth D. Mandl, Abla Mawudeku, Gunther Eysenbach, and John S. Brownstein. "Use of Unstructured Event-Based Reports for Global Infectious Disease Surveillance." *Emerging Infectious Diseases* 15, no. 5 (May 2009): 689–95. https://doi.org/10.3201/eid1505.081114.

Kent, Sherman. "Words of Estimative Probability." *Studies in Intelligence* 8, no. 4 (1964): 49–65.

Keshaviah, Aparna, Xindi C. Hu, and Henry Marisa. "Developing a Flexible National Wastewater Surveillance System for COVID-19 and Beyond." *Environmental Health Perspectives* 129, no. 4 (2021): 045002. https://doi.org/10.1289/EHP8572.

Khor, Swee Kheng, and David L. Heymann. "Pandemic Preparedness in the 21st Century: Which Way Forward?" *Lancet Public Health* 6, no. 6 (June 1, 2021): e357–58. https://doi.org/10.1016/S2468-2667(21)00101-8.

Kim, Pan Suk. "South Korea's Fast Response to Coronavirus Disease: Implications on Public Policy and Public Management Theory." *Public Management Review* 23, no. 12 (2021): 1736–47. https://doi.org/10.1080/14719037.2020.1766266.

Kim, Sun, and Marcia C. Castro. "Spatiotemporal Pattern of COVID-19 and Government Response in South Korea (as of May 31, 2020)." *International Journal of Infectious Diseases* 98 (September 1, 2020): 328–33. https://doi.org/10.1016/j.ijid.2020.07.004.

Klain, Ronald. "Confronting the Pandemic Threat." *Democracy* 40 (Spring 2016). https://democracyjournal.org/magazine/40/confronting-the-pandemic-threat/.

Koblentz, Gregory D. *Living Weapons: Biological Warfare and International Security.* Ithaca, NY: Cornell University Press, 2009.

Koblentz, Gregory D., and Stevie Kiesel. "The COVID-19 Pandemic: Catalyst or Complication for Bioterrorism?" *Studies in Conflict & Terrorism*, July 14, 2021, 1–27. https://doi.org/10.1080/1057610X.2021.1944023.

Kogan, Nicole E., Leonardo Clemente, Parker Liautaud, Justin Kaashoek, Nicholas B. Link, Andre T. Nguyen, Fred S. Lu, et al. "An Early Warning Approach to Monitor COVID-19 Activity with Multiple Digital Traces in Near Real Time." *Science Advances* 7, no. 10 (March 1, 2021): eabd6989. https://doi.org/10.1126/sciadv.abd6989.

Kpozehouen, Elizabeth Benedict, Xin Chen, Mengyao Zhu, and C. Raina Macintyre. "Using Open-Source Intelligence to Detect Early Signals of COVID-19 in China: Descriptive Study." *JMIR Public Health Surveillance* 6, no. 3 (September 18, 2020): e18939. https://doi.org/10.2196/18939.

Lakoff, Andrew. "From Population to Vital System: National Security and the Changing Object of Public Health." In *Biosecurity Interventions*, edited by Andrew Lakoff and Stephen Collier, 33–60. New York: Columbia University Press, 2008. https://doi.org/10.7312/lako14606-002.

———. "Two Regimes of Global Health." *Humanity* 1, no. 1 (Fall 2010): 59–79.

Langmuir, Alexander D. "Communicable Disease Surveillance: Evolution of the Concept of Surveillance in the United States." *Proceedings of the Royal Society of Medicine* 64 (June 1971): 681–84.

———. "Developing Concepts in Surveillance." *Milbank Memorial Fund Quarterly* 43, no. 2 pt. 2 (April 1965): 369–72.

———. "The Epidemic Intelligence Service of the Center for Disease Control." *Public Health Reports* 95, no. 5 (1980): 470–77.

———. "The Surveillance of Communicable Diseases of National Importance." *New England Journal of Medicine* 268, no. 4 (January 24, 1963): 182–92. https://doi.org /10.1056/NEJM196301242680405.

Lankford, Ana Maria, Derrick Storzieri, and Joseph Fitsanakis. "Spies and the Virus: The COVID-19 Pandemic and Intelligence Communication in the United States." *Frontiers in Communication* 5 (2020): 1–11. https://doi.org/10.3389/fcomm.2020 .582245.

Laqueur, Walter. "The Question of Judgment: Intelligence and Medicine." *Journal of Contemporary History* 18, no. 4 (1983): 533–48.

Lawrence, Susan V. "COVID-19 and China: A Chronology of Events (December 2019-January 2020)." Congressional Research Service, May 13, 2020. https://crs reports.congress.gov/product/pdf/r/r46354.

Lazer, David, Ryan Kennedy, Gary King, and Alessandro Vespignani. "The Parable of Google Flu: Traps in Big Data Analysis." *Science* 343, no. 6176 (March 14, 2014): 1203–5. https://doi.org/10.1126/science.1248506.

Lee, Kelley. Review of "The Health of Nations: Infectious Disease, Environmental Change, and Their Effects on National Security and Development." *BMJ: British Medical Journal* 324, no. 7338 (March 16, 2002): 683. https://www.ncbi.nlm.nih.gov /pmc/articles/PMC1122610/.

Lee, Kelley, and Julianne Piper. "Reviving the Role of GPHIN in Global Epidemic Intelligence." In *Stress Tested: The COVID-19 Pandemic and Canadian National Security*, edited by Leah West, Thomas Juneau, and Amarnath Amarasingam, 177–91. Calgary, Alberta: University of Calgary Press, 2021.

Lentzos, Filippa, Michael S. Goodman, and James M. Wilson. "Health Security Intelligence: Engaging across Disciplines and Sectors." *Intelligence and National Security* 35, no. 4 (June 6, 2020): 465–76. https://doi.org/10.1080/02684527.2020.1750166.

Levy, Barry S., and Victor W. Sidel, eds. *War and Public Health.* 2d ed. Oxford: Oxford University Press, 2008.

Li, Cuilian, Li Jia Chen, Xueyu Chen, Mingzhi Zhang, Chi Pui Pang, and Haoyu Chen. "Retrospective Analysis of the Possibility of Predicting the COVID-19 Outbreak from Internet Searches and Social Media Data, China, 2020." *Eurosurveillance* 25, no. 10 (2020). https://doi.org/10.2807/1560-7917.ES.2020.25.10.2000199.

Lopreite, Milena, Pietro Panzarasa, Michelangelo Puliga, and Massimo Riccaboni. "Early Warnings of COVID-19 Outbreaks across Europe from Social Media?" arXiv .org, December 2020. https://EconPapers.repec.org/RePEc:arx:papers:2008.02649.

Lowenthal, Mark M. "Grant vs. Sherman: Paradoxes of Intelligence and Combat Leadership." In *Paradoxes of Strategic Intelligence: Essays in Honor of Michael I. Handel*, edited by Richard K. Betts and Thomas G. Mahnken, 190–202. New York: Routledge, 2003.

———. *Intelligence: From Secrets to Policy.* 8th ed. Thousand Oaks, CA: CQ, 2020.

———. "Towards a Reasonable Standard for Analysis: How Right, How Often on Which Issues?." *Intelligence and National Security* 23, no. 3 (June 1, 2008): 303–15. https:// doi.org/10.1080/02684520802121190.

Lo Yuk-ping, Catherine, and Nicholas Thomas. "How Is Health a Security Issue?: Politics, Responses and Issues." *Health Policy and Planning* 25, no. 6 (November 1, 2010): 447–53. https://doi.org/10.1093/heapol/czq063.

Lyon, Regan F. "The COVID-19 Response Has Uncovered and Increased Our Vulnerability to Biological Warfare." *Military Medicine* 186, no. 7–8 (July 1, 2021): 193–96. https://doi.org/10.1093/milmed/usab061.

Lyseen, A. K., C. Nøhr, E. M. Sørensen, O. Gudes, E. M. Geraghty, N. T. Shaw, C. Bivona-Tellez, and IMIA Health GIS Working Group. "A Review and Framework for Categorizing Current Research and Development in Health Related Geographical Information Systems (GIS) Studies." *Yearbook of Medical Informatics* 9, no. 1 (August 15, 2014): 110–24. https://doi.org/10.15265/IY-2014-0 008.

Maclean, Sandra J. "Microbes, Mad Cows and Militaries: Exploring the Links Between Health and Security." *Security Dialogue* 39, no. 5 (October 1, 2008): 475–94. https://doi.org/10.1177/0967010608096149.

Magid, Avi, Anat Gesser-Edelsburg, and Manfred S. Green. "The Role of Informal Digital Surveillance Systems Before, During and After Infectious Disease Outbreaks: A Critical Analysis." In *Defence Against Bioterrorism: Methods for Prevention and Control*, edited by Vladan Radosavljevic, Ines Banjari, and Goran Belojevic, 189–201. New York: Springer, 2018. https://doi.org/10.1007/978-94-024-1263-5_14.

Marrin, Stephen. "Why Strategic Intelligence Analysis Has Limited Influence on American Foreign Policy." *Intelligence and National Security* 32, no. 6 (September 19, 2017): 725–42. https://doi.org/10.1080/02684527.2016.1275139.

Marrin, Stephen, and Jonathan D. Clemente. "Improving Intelligence Analysis by Looking to the Medical Profession." *International Journal of Intelligence and CounterIntelligence* 18, no. 4 (December 1, 2005): 707–29. https://doi.org/10.1080/08850600 590945434.

Martin, Javier, Dimitra Klapsa, Thomas Wilton, Maria Zambon, Emma Bentley, Erika Bujaki, Martin Fritzsche, Ryan Mate, and Manasi Majumdar. "Tracking SARS-CoV-2 in Sewage: Evidence of Changes in Virus Variant Predominance during COVID-19 Pandemic." *Viruses* 12, no. 10 (2020). https://doi.org/10.3390/v12101144.

Mathews, Jessica Tuchman. "Redefining Security." *Foreign Affairs* 68, no. 2 (Spring 1989): 162–77.

McClellan, Mark, Scott Gottlieb, Farzad Mostashari, Caitlin Rivers, and Lauren Silvis. "A National COVID-19 Surveillance System: Achieving Containment." Washington, DC: Duke-Margolis Health Policy Center, April 7, 2020. https://healthpolicy.duke.edu/publications/national-covid-19-surveillance-system-achieving-containment.

McDermott, Rose. "The Use and Abuse of Medical Intelligence." *Intelligence and National Security* 22, no. 4 (August 2007): 491–520.

McInnes, Colin, and Anne Roemer-Mahler. "From Security to Risk: Reframing Global Health Threats." *International Affairs* 93, no. 6 (November 1, 2017): 1313–37. https://doi.org/10.1093/ia/iix187.

McNabb, Scott J. N., Stella Chungong, Mike Ryan, Tadesse Wuhib, Peter Nsubuga, Wondi Alemu, Vilma Carande-Kulis, and Guenael Rodier. "Conceptual Framework of Public Health Surveillance and Action and Its Application in Health Sector Reform." *BMC Public Health* 2, no. 1 (January 29, 2002): 2. https://doi.org/10.1186/1471-2458-2-2.

McNabb, Scott J. N., J. Mark Conde, Lisa Ferland, William MacWright, Ziad A. Memish, Stacy Okutani, Meeyoung M. Park, Paige Ryland, Affan T. Shaikh, and Vivek Singh, eds. *Transforming Public Health Surveillance: Proactive Measures for Prevention, Detection, and Response*. Amman, Jordan: Elsevier, 2016.

Michaud, Joshua. "National Center for Medical Intelligence." In *Encyclopedia of Bioterrorism Defense*, 2nd. ed., edited by Rebecca Katz and Raymond A. Zilinskas, 1–3. Hoboken, NJ: Wiley, 2011.

Migliore, Laurie, Dawnkimberly Hopkins, Savannah Jumpp, Ceferina Brackett, and Jessica Cromheecke. "Medical Intelligence Team Lessons Learned: Early Activation and Knowledge Product Development Mitigate COVID-19 Threats." *Military Medicine* 186, no. 2 (September 1, 2021): 15–22. https://doi.org/10.1093/milmed /usab190.

Miller, David. "The US Defense Intelligence Agency's National Center for Medical Intelligence." *Journal of the Royal Naval Medical Service* 95, no. 2 (2009): 89–91.

Miller, Seumas, and Marcus Smith. "Ethics, Public Health and Technology Responses to COVID-19." *Bioethics* 35, no. 4 (May 1, 2021): 366–71. https://doi.org/10.1111 /bioe.12856.

Mina, Michael J., C. Jessica E. Metcalf, Adrian B. McDermott, Daniel C. Douek, Jeremy Farrar, and Bryan T. Grenfell. "A Global Immunological Observatory to Meet a Time of Pandemics." *ELife* 9 (June 8, 2020): 1–5. https://doi.org/10.7554/eLife.58989.

Montgomery, Joel M., Abbey Woolverton, Sarah Hedges, Dana Pitts, Jessica Alexander, Kashef Ijaz, Fred Angulo, Scott Dowell, Rebecca Katz, and Olga Henao. "Ten Years of Global Disease Detection and Counting: Program Accomplishments and Lessons Learned in Building Global Health Security." *BMC Public Health* 19, no. 3 (May 10, 2019): 1–9. https://doi.org/10.1186/s12889-019-6769-2.

Monti, Mario, Aleksandra Torbica, Elias Mossialos, and Martin McKee. "A New Strategy for Health and Sustainable Development in the Light of the COVID-19 Pandemic." *Lancet* 398, no. 10305 (September 18, 2021): 1029–31. https://doi.org/10 .1016/S0140-6736(21)01995-4.

Moon, Suerie, Devi Sridhar, Muhammad A. Pate, Ashish K. Jha, Chelsea Clinton, Sophie Delaunay, Valnora Edwin, et al. "Will Ebola Change the Game?: Ten Essential Reforms before the Next Pandemic." Report of the Harvard-LSHTM Independent Panel on the Global Response to Ebola. *Lancet* 386, no. 10009 (November 28, 2015): 2204–21. https://doi.org/10.1016/S0140-6736(15)00946-0.

Moore, Melinda, Gail Fisher, and Clare Stevens. "Toward Integrated DoD Biosurveillance: Assessment and Opportunities." Santa Monica, CA: RAND, 2013. https:// www.rand.org/pubs/research_reports/RR399.html.

Morgan, Oliver W., Ximena Aguilera, Andrea Ammon, John Amuasi, Ibrahima Socé Fall, Tom Frieden, David Heymann, et al. "Disease Surveillance for the COVID-19 Era: Time for Bold Changes." *Lancet* 397, no. 10292 (June 19, 2021): 2317–19. https://doi.org/10.1016/S0140-6736(21)01096-5.

Morse, Stephen S. "Global Infectious Disease Surveillance and Health Intelligence." *Health Affairs* 26, no. 4 (August 2007): 1069–77.

———. "Public Health Surveillance and Infectious Disease Detection." *Biosecurity and Bioterrorism: Biodefense Strategy, Practice, and Science* 10, no. 1 (March 28, 2012): 6–16. https://www.liebertpub.com/doi/10.1089/bsp.2011.0088?url_ver=Z39.88-2003 &rfr_id=ori:rid:crossref.org&rfr_dat=cr_pub%20%200pubmed.

Murray, Jillian, and Adam L. Cohen. "Infectious Disease Surveillance." In *International Encyclopedia of Public Health*, 2nd. ed., edited by Stella R. Quah, 222–29. Oxford: Academic Press, 2017. https://doi.org/10.1016/B978-0-12-803678-5.00517-8.

Myers, Jennifer F., Robert E. Snyder, Charsey Cole Porse, Selam Tecle, and Phil Lowenthal. "Identification and Monitoring of International Travelers During the Initial

Phase of an Outbreak of COVID-19—California, February 3–March 17, 2020." *MMWR: Morbidity and Mortality Weekly Report* 69, no. 19 (May 15, 2020): 599–602.

Mykhalovskiy, E., and L. Weir. "The Global Public Health Intelligence Network and Early Warning Outbreak Detection—A Canadian Contribution to Global Public Health." *Canadian Journal of Public Health* 97, no. 1 (February 2006): 42–44. https://doi.org /10.1007/BF03405213.

Nash, Denis, and Elvin Geng. "Goal-Aligned, Epidemic Intelligence for the Public Health Response to the COVID-19 Pandemic." *American Journal of Public Health* 110, no. 8 (July 2, 2020): 1154–56. https://doi.org/10.2105/AJPH.2020.305794.

National Center for Medical Intelligence. "Worldwide: New 2009-H1N1 Influenza Virus Poses Potential Threat to U.S. Forces." Defense Intelligence Assessment, May 1, 2009. https://www.globalsecurity.org/security/library/report/2009/090501 -di-1812-1544-09.pdf.

National Biosurveillance Advisory Subcommittee. "Improving the Nation's Ability to Detect and Respond to 21st Century Urgent Health Threats: First Report of the National Biosurveillance Advisory Subcommittee." April 2009. https://stacks.cdc .gov/view/cdc/12000.

Neustadt, Richard E., and Harvey V. Fineberg. *The Swine Flu Affair: Decision-Making on a Slippery Disease.* Washington, DC: National Academies Press, 2009.

NIC (National Intelligence Council). "Climate Change and International Responses Increasing Challenges to US National Security through 2040." National Intelligence Estimate, October 2021. https://www.dni.gov/index.php/newsroom/reports -publications/reports-publications-2021/item/2253-national-intelligence-estimate -on-climate-change.

———. "The Global Infectious Disease Threat and Its Implications for the United States." January 2000. https://www.dni.gov/files/documents/infectiousdiseases_2000.pdf.

———. "Global Trends: Paradox of Progress." January 2017. https://www.dni.gov/index .php/global-trends-home.

———. "Global Trends 2025: A Transformed World." November 2008. https://www.dni .gov/files/documents/Newsroom/Reports%20and%20Pubs/2025_Global_Trends _Final_Report.pdf.

———. "Global Trends 2030: Alternative Worlds." December 2012. https://www.dni.gov /files/documents/GlobalTrends_2030.pdf.

———. "Global Trends 2040: A More Contested World." March 2021. https://www.dni .gov/files/ODNI/documents/assessments/GlobalTrends_2040.pdf.

———. "Mapping the Global Future: Report of the National Intelligence Council's 2020 Project." December 2004. https://www.odni.gov/files/documents/Global%20 Trends_Mapping%20the%20Global%20Future%202020%20Project.pdf.

———. "The Next Wave of HIV/AIDS: Nigeria, Ethiopia, Russia, India, and China." September 2002. https://www.dni.gov/files/documents/Special%20Report_The% 20Next%20Wave%20of%20HIV_AIDS.pdf.

———. "SARS: Down but Still a Threat." August 2003. https://apps.dtic.mil/sti/pdfs /ADA511659.pdf.

———. "Strategic Implications of Global Health." December 2008. https://www.dni.gov /files/documents/Special%20Report_ICA%20Global%20Health%202008.pdf.

9/11 Commission. *The 9/11 Commission Report: Final Report of the National Commission on Terrorism Attacks upon the United States.* Authorized ed. New York: W. W. Norton, 2004.

Nuzzo, Jennifer B. "To Stop a Pandemic: A Better Approach to Global Health Security." *Foreign Affairs* 100, no. 1 (February 2021): 36–42.

Nuzzo, Jennifer B., and Gigi Kwik Gronvall. "Achieving the Right Balance in Governance of Public Health Surveillance." In *Transforming Public Health Surveillance: Proactive Measures for Prevention, Detection, and Response,* edited by Scott J. N. McNabb et al., 169–78. Amman, Jordan: Elsevier, 2016.

Omand, David, Jamie Bartlett, and Carl Miller. "Introducing Social Media Intelligence (SOCMINT)." *Intelligence and National Security* 27, no. 6 (December 1, 2012): 801–23. https://doi.org/10.1080/02684527.2012.716965.

Oppenheimer, Michael. "As the World Burns: Climate Change's Dangerous Next Phase." *Foreign Affairs* 99, no. 6 (December 2020): 34–40.

O'Shea, Jesse. "Digital Disease Detection: A Systematic Review of Event-Based Internet Biosurveillance Systems." *International Journal of Medical Informatics* 101 (May 2017): 15–22. https://doi.org/10.1016/j.ijmedinf.2017.01.019.

Ostergard, Robert L. "The West Africa Ebola Outbreak (2014–2016): A Health Intelligence Failure?." *Intelligence and National Security* 35, no. 4 (June 6, 2020): 477–92. https://doi.org/10.1080/02684527.2020.1750136.

Osterholm, Michael T. "Preparing for the Next Pandemic." *Foreign Affairs* 84, no. 4 (August 2005): 24–37.

Osterholm, Michael T., and Mark Olshaker. "Chronicle of a Pandemic Foretold." *Foreign Affairs* 99, no. 4 (August 2020).

Park, Meeyoung M., and Lauren Reeves. "Models of Public Health Surveillance." In *Transforming Public Health Surveillance: Proactive Measures for Prevention, Detection, and Response,* edited by Scott J. N. McNabb et al., 32–49. Amman, Jordan: Elsevier, 2016.

Pei, Sen, Sasikiran Kandula, and Jeffrey Shaman. "Differential Effects of Intervention Timing on COVID-19 Spread in the United States." *Science Advances* 6, no. 49 (December 4, 2020): 1–9. https://doi.org/10.1126/sciadv.abd6370.

Pei, Sen, Xian Teng, Paul Lewis, and Jeffrey Shaman. "Optimizing Respiratory Virus Surveillance Networks Using Uncertainty Propagation." *Nature Communications* 12, no. 1 (January 11, 2021): 1–10. https://doi.org/10.1038/s41467-020-20399-3.

Pekar, Jonathan E., Andrew Magee, Edyth Parker, Niema Moshiri, Katherine Izhikevich, Jennifer L. Havens, Karthik Gangavarapu, et al. "Sars-Cov-2 Emergence Very Likely Resulted from at Least Two Zoonotic Events." Zenodo, February 26, 2022. https://doi.org/10.5281/zenodo.6342616.

Pellerin, Cheryl. "Medical Intelligence Center Monitors Health Threats." *American Forces Press Service,* October 10, 2012. https://www.dni.gov/index.php/newsroom/news-articles/ic-in-the-news-2012/item/739-medical-intelligence-center-monitors-health-threats.

Peterson, Susan. "Epidemic Disease and National Security." *Security Studies* 12, no. 2 (December 1, 2002): 43–81. https://doi.org/10.1080/09636410212120009.

———. "Global Health and Security: Reassessing the Links." In *The Oxford Handbook of International Security.* Cambridge: Oxford University Press, 2018. www.oxfordhandbooks.com.

Petitjean, Mirielle M. "Intelligence Support to Disaster Relief and Humanitarian Assistance." *Intelligencer* 10, no. 3 (Winter-Spring 2013): 57–60.

Poland, Gregory A. "Another Coronavirus, Another Epidemic, Another Warning." *Vaccine* 38, no. 10 (February 28, 2020): v–vi. https://doi.org/10.1016/j.vaccine.2020.02.039.

Polyak, Marat G., Jane Blake, Jeff Collmann, and James M. Wilson. "Emergence of Severe Acute Respiratory Syndrome (SARS) in the People's Republic of China, 2002–2003: A Case Study to Define Requirements for Detection and Assessment of International Biological Threats." Washington, DC: Georgetown University Medical Center, n.d.

Price-Smith, Andrew T. *Contagion and Chaos: Disease, Ecology, and National Security in the Era of Globalization.* Cambridge, MA: MIT Press, 2009.

———. *The Health of Nations: Infectious Disease, Environmental Change, and Their Effects on National Security and Development.* Cambridge, MA: MIT Press, 2002.

Rahim, M., B. Kazi, K. Bile, M. Munir, and A. R. Khan. "The Impact of the Disease Early Warning System in Responding to Natural Disasters and Conflict Crises in Pakistan." *Eastern Mediterranean Health Journal=La Revue de Sante de La Mediterranee Orientale=Al-Majallah al-Sihhiyah Li-Sharq al-Mutawassit* 16 (2010): S114–21.

Reingold, Arthur. "If Syndromic Surveillance Is the Answer, What Is the Question?." *Biosecurity and Bioterrorism: Biodefense Strategy, Practice, and Science* 1, no. 2 (June 1, 2003): 77–81. https://doi.org/10.1089/153871303766275745.

Rolka, Henry, and Kara Contreary. "Past Contributions." In *Transforming Public Health Surveillance: Proactive Measures for Prevention, Detection, and Response*, edited by Scott J. N. McNabb et al., 13–23. Amman, Jordan: Elsevier, 2016.

Rushton, Simon. "Global Health Security: Security for Whom? Security from What?." *Political Studies* 59, no. 4 (November 7, 2011): 779–96. https://doi.org/10.1111/j.1467-9248.2011.00919.x.

———. *Security and Public Health: Pandemics and Politics in the Contemporary World.* Cambridge, UK: Polity, 2019.

Rushton, Simon, and Jeremy Youde, eds. *Routledge Handbook of Global Health Security.* London: Routledge Handbooks Online, 2015. https://www.taylorfrancis.com/books/9781138501973.

Russell, Kevin L. "Contributions of the United States Military Public Health Surveillance to Global Public Health Security." In *Transforming Public Health Surveillance: Proactive Measures for Prevention, Detection, and Response*, edited by Scott J. N. McNabb et al., 206–22. Amman, Jordan: Elsevier, 2016.

Russell, Kevin L., Jennifer Rubenstein, Ronald L. Burke, Kelly G. Vest, Matthew C. Johns, Jose L. Sanchez, William Meyer, Mark M. Fukuda, and David L. Blazes. "The Global Emerging Infection Surveillance and Response System (GEIS), a U.S. Government Tool for Improved Global Biosurveillance: A Review of 2009." *BMC Public Health* 11, Suppl 2 (March 4, 2011): 1–10. https://doi.org/10.1186/1471-2458-11-S2-S2.

Saran, Sameer, Priyanka Singh, Vishal Kumar, and Prakash Chauhan. "Review of Geospatial Technology for Infectious Disease Surveillance: Use Case on COVID-19." *Journal of the Indian Society of Remote Sensing*, August 18, 2020, 1–18. https://doi.org/10.1007/s12524-020-01140-5.

Schaffner, William, and F. Marc LaForce. "Training Field Epidemiologists: Alexander D. Langmuir and the Epidemic Intelligence Service." *American Journal of Epidemiology* 144, no. 8 (1996): S16–S22.

Schneider, Eric C. "Failing the Test—The Tragic Data Gap Undermining the U.S. Pandemic Response." *New England Journal of Medicine* 383, no. 4 (May 15, 2020): 299–302. https://doi.org/10.1056/NEJMp2014836.

Sheel, Meru, Julie Collins, Mike Kama, Devina Nand, Daniel Faktaufon, Josaia Samuela, Viema Biaukula, et al. "Evaluation of the Early Warning, Alert and Response System after Cyclone Winston, Fiji, 2016." *Bulletin of the World Health Organization* 97, no. 3 (March 1, 2019): 178–189C. https://www.ncbi.nlm.nih.gov/pmc/articles /PMC6453321/pdf/BLT.18.211409.pdf.

Shelton, John. "International Health and Intelligence Gathering: One in the Same or Rival Factions?." *Journal of Biosecurity, Biosafety and Biodefense Law* 2, no. 1 (March 2, 2012): 1–21.

Sidel, Victor W., and Barry S. Levy. "War, Terrorism, and Public Health." *Journal of Law, Medicine & Ethics* 31, no. 4 (December 1, 2003): 516–23. https://doi.org/10.1111/j .1748-720X.2003.tb00119.x.

Singh, Sudhvir, Christine McNab, Rose McKeon Olson, Nellie Bristol, Cody Nolan, Elin Bergstrøm, Michael Bartos, et al. "How an Outbreak Became a Pandemic: A Chronological Analysis of Crucial Junctures and International Obligations in the Early Months of the COVID-19 Pandemic." *Lancet* 398, no. 10316 (December 4, 2021): 2109–24. https://doi.org/10.1016/S0140-6736(21)01897-3.

Smith, Marcus, and Patrick Walsh. "Improving Health Security and Intelligence Capabilities to Mitigate Biological Threats." *International Journal of Intelligence, Security, and Public Affairs* 23, no. 2 (May 4, 2021): 139–55. https://doi.org/10.1080 /23800992.2021.1953826.

Stoto, Michael A., and Melissa A. Higdon, eds. *The Public Health Response to 2009 H1N1: A Systems Perspective.* Oxford: Oxford University Press, 2015.

Stoto, Michael A., and Ying Zhang. "Did Advances in Global Surveillance and Notification Systems Make a Difference in the 2009 H1N1 Pandemic?." In *The Public Health Response to 2009 H1N1: A Systems Perspective,* edited by Michael A. Stoto and Melissa A. Higdon, 19–39. Oxford: Oxford University Press, 2015.

Summers, Jennifer, Hao-Yuan Cheng, Hsien-Ho Lin, Lucy Telfar Barnard, Amanda Kvalsvig, Nick Wilson, and Michael G. Baker. "Potential Lessons from the Taiwan and New Zealand Health Responses to the COVID-19 Pandemic." *Lancet Regional Health—Western Pacific* 4 (October 21, 2020). https://doi.org/10.1016/j.lanwpc .2020.100044.

Sun, Nina. "Applying Siracusa: A Call for a General Comment on Public Health Emergencies." *Health and Human Rights* 22, no. 1 (June 2020): 387–90.

Tarantola, Daniel, and Nabarun Dasgupta. "COVID-19 Surveillance Data: A Primer for Epidemiology and Data Science." *American Journal of Public Health* 111, no. 4 (April 1, 2021): 614–19. https://doi.org/10.2105/AJPH.2020.306088.

Taylor, Allyn L., Roojin Habibi, Gian Luca Burci, Stephanie Dagron, Mark Eccleston-Turner, Lawrence O. Gostin, Benjamin Mason Meier, et al. "Solidarity in the Wake of COVID-19: Reimagining the International Health Regulations." *Lancet* 396, no. 10244 (July 11, 2020): 82–83. https://doi.org/10.1016/S0140-6736(20)31417-3.

Thacker, Stephen B., Judith R. Qualters, and Lisa M. Lee. "Public Health Surveillance in the United States: Evolution and Challenges." *MMWR Suppl* 61 (July 27, 2012): 3–9.

Toner, Eric S., and Jennifer B. Nuzzo. "Acting on the Lessons of SARS: What Remains to Be Done?." *Biosecurity and Bioterrorism: Biodefense Strategy, Practice, and Science* 9, no. 2 (May 25, 2011): 169–74. https://doi.org/10.1089/bsp.2010.0074.

Toner, Eric S., Jennifer B. Nuzzo, Matthew Watson, Crystal Franco, Tara Kirk Sell, Anita Cicero, and Thomas V. Inglesby. "Biosurveillance Where It Happens: State and Local Capabilities and Needs." *Biosecurity and Bioterrorism: Biodefense Strategy, Practice, and Science* 9, no. 4 (September 9, 2011): 321–30. https://doi.org/10.1089 /bsp.2011.0049.

Tromblay, Darren E. "Botching Bio-Surveillance: The Department of Homeland Security and COVID-19 Pandemic." *International Journal of Intelligence and Counter-Intelligence* 35, no. 1 (January 2, 2022): 164–67. https://doi.org/10.1080/08850607.2021.1888035.

Tsao, Daniel. "Psychiatrists, Professors, Patriots: Drs. Jerrold Post (1934–2020) and Laurence Cove (1933–2020)." *Studies in Intelligence* 65, no. 1 (March 2021): 3–5.

Tulchinsky, Theodore H. "John Snow, Cholera, the Broad Street Pump; Waterborne Diseases Then and Now." *Case Studies in Public Health*, 2018, 77–99. https://doi.org/10.1016/B978-0-12-804571-8.00017-2.

Udugama, Buddhisha, Pranav Kadhiresan, Hannah N. Kozlowski, Ayden Malekjahani, Matthew Osborne, Vanessa Y. C. Li, Hongmin Chen, Samira Mubareka, Jonathan B. Gubbay, and Warren C. W. Chan. "Diagnosing COVID-19: The Disease and Tools for Detection." *ACS Nano* 14, no. 4 (April 28, 2020): 3822–35. https://doi.org/10.1021/acsnano.0c02624.

UK Government Cabinet Office. "National Security Strategy and Strategic Defence and Security Review 2015." London: Cabinet Office, November 2015. https://assets.publishing.service.gov.uk/government/uploads/system/uploads/attachment_data/file/478936/52309_Cm_9161_NSS_SD_Review_PRINT_only.pdf.

UK Ministry of Defence. "Global Strategic Trends: The Future Starts Today." 6th ed. London: Ministry of Defence, 2018. https://www.gov.uk/government/publications/global-strategic-trends.

Ullman, Richard H. "Redefining Security." *International Security* 8, no. 1 (1983): 129–53. https://doi.org/10.2307/2538489.

Van Puyvelde, Damien. "Fusing Drug Enforcement: A Study of the El Paso Intelligence Center." *Intelligence and National Security* 31, no. 6 (September 18, 2016): 888–902. https://doi.org/10.1080/02684527.2015.1100373.

Velikina, Rita, Virginia Dato, and Michael M. Wagner. "Governmental Public Health." In *Handbook of Biosurveillance*, edited by Michael M. Wagner et al., 67–87. San Diego, CA: Elsevier Science & Technology, 2006.

Velsko, Stephan, and Thomas Bates. "A Conceptual Architecture for National Biosurveillance: Moving Beyond Situational Awareness to Enable Digital Detection of Emerging Threats." *Health Security* 14, no. 3 (June 1, 2016): 189–201. https://doi.org/10.1089/hs.2015.0063.

Vinuales, Jorge, Suerie Moon, Ginevra Le Moli, and Gian-Luca Burci. "A Global Pandemic Treaty Should Aim for Deep Prevention." *Lancet* 397, no. 10287 (May 15, 2021): 1791–92. https://doi.org/10.1016/S0140-6736(21)00948-X.

Vlieg, Willemijn L., Ewout B. Fanoy, Liselotte van Asten, Xiaobo Liu, Jun Yang, Eva Pilot, Paul Bijkerk, et al. "Comparing National Infectious Disease Surveillance Systems: China and the Netherlands." *BMC Public Health* 17, no. 415 (May 8, 2017): 1–9. https://doi.org/10.1186/s12889-017-4319-3.

Vogel, Kathleen M. "Intelligent Assessment: Putting Emerging Biotechnology Threats in Context." *Bulletin of the Atomic Scientists* 69, no. 1 (January 1, 2013): 43–52. https://doi.org/10.1177/0096340212470813.

Wagner, Michael M. "Methods for Evaluating Surveillance Data." In *Handbook of Biosurveillance*, edited by Michael M. Wagner et al., 313–19. San Diego, CA: Elsevier Science & Technology, 2006.

Wagner, Michael M., Andrew W. Moore, and Ron M Aryel, eds. *Handbook of Biosurveillance*. San Diego, CA: Elsevier Science & Technology, 2006. http://ebookcentral.proquest.com/lib/ebook-nps/detail.action?docID=270232.

Walsh, Patrick F. "Improving 'Five Eyes' Health Security Intelligence Capabilities: Leadership and Governance Challenges." *Intelligence and National Security* 35, no. 4 (June 6, 2020): 586–602. https://doi.org/10.1080/02684527.2020.1750156.

———. *Intelligence, Biosecurity and Bioterrorism*. London: Palgrave Macmillan, 2018.

———. "Managing Emerging Health Security Threats Since 9/11: The Role of Intelligence." *International Journal of Intelligence and CounterIntelligence* 29, no. 2 (April 2, 2016): 341–67. https://doi.org/10.1080/08850607.2016.1121048.

Wang, C. Jason, Chun Y. Ng, and Robert H. Brook. "Response to COVID-19 in Taiwan: Big Data Analytics, New Technology, and Proactive Testing." *JAMA* 323, no. 14 (April 14, 2020): 1341–42. https://doi.org/10.1001/jama.2020.3151.

Wang, Wenjun, Yikai Wang, Xin Zhang, Xiaoli Jia, Yaping Li, and Shuangsuo Dang. "Using WeChat, a Chinese Social Media App, for Early Detection of the COVID-19 Outbreak in December 2019: Retrospective Study." *JMIR MHealth and UHealth* 8, no. 10 (October 5, 2020): e19589. https://doi.org/10.2196/19589.

Watsa, Mrinalini. "Rigorous Wildlife Disease Surveillance." *Science* 369, no. 6500 (July 10, 2020): 145. https://doi.org/10.1126/science.abc0017.

Wenham, Clare. "Digitalizing Disease Surveillance: The Global Safety Net?." *Global Health Governance* 10, no. 2 (Fall 2016). http://blogs.shu.edu/ghg/2016/10/16/digitalizing-disease-surveillance-the-global-safety-net/.

———. "GPHIN, GOARN, GONE?: The Role of the World Health Organization in Global Disease Surveillance and Response." In *The Politics of Surveillance and Response to Disease Outbreaks*, edited by Sara E. Davies and Jeremy R. Youde, 107–19. Farnham, UK: Ashgate, 2015.

Whipple, Chris. *The Spymasters: How the CIA Directors Shape History and the Future*. New York: Scribner, 2020.

White House. "Executive Order on Organizing and Mobilizing the United States Government to Provide a Unified and Effective Response to Combat COVID-19 and to Provide United States Leadership on Global Health and Security." January 20, 2021. https://www.whitehouse.gov/briefing-room/presidential-actions/2021/01/20/executive-order-organizing-and-mobilizing-united-states-government-to-provide-unified-and-effective-response-to-combat-covid-19-and-to-provide-united-states-leadership-on-global-health-and-security/.

———. "Interim National Security Strategic Guidance." March 2021. https://www.whitehouse.gov/wp-content/uploads/2021/03/NSC-1v2.pdf.

———. "National Security Memorandum on United States Global Leadership to Strengthen the International COVID-19 Response and to Advance Global Health Security and Biological Preparedness." January 21, 2021. https://www.whitehouse.gov/briefing-room/statements-releases/2021/01/21/national-security-directive-united-states-global-leadership-to-strengthen-the-international-covid-19-response-and-to-advance-global-health-security-and-biological-preparedness/.

———. "National Security Presidential Directive-1: Organization of the National Security Council System." February 13, 2001. https://fas.org/irp/offdocs/nspd/nspd-1.pdf.

———. "National Security Strategy." May 2010. https://obamawhitehouse.archives.gov/sites/default/files/rss_viewer/national_security_strategy.pdf.

———. "National Strategy for Biosurveillance." July 2012. https://obamawhitehouse.archives.gov/sites/default/files/National_Strategy_for_Biosurveillance_July_2012.pdf.

———. "National Strategy for the COVID-19 Response and Pandemic Preparedness." January 2021. https://www.whitehouse.gov/wp-content/uploads/2021/01/National-Strategy-for-the-COVID-19-Response-and-Pandemic-Preparedness.pdf.

———. "Presidential Decision Directive NSTC-7, Emerging Infectious Diseases." June 12, 1996. https://fas.org/irp/offdocs/pdd/pdd-nstc-7.pdf.

———. "Remarks by President Obama in Address to the United Nations General Assembly." September 21, 2011. https://obamawhitehouse.archives.gov/the-press-office/2011/09/21/remarks-president-obama-address-united-nations-general-assembly.

Wibulpolprasert, Suwit, and Mushtaque Chowdhury. "World Health Organization: Overhaul or Dismantle?." *American Journal of Public Health* 106, no. 11 (November 2016): 1910–11. https://doi.org/10.2105/AJPH.2016.303469.

Wilburn, Jennifer, Catherine O'Connor, Amanda L. Walsh, and Dilys Morgan. "Identifying Potential Emerging Threats through Epidemic Intelligence Activities—Looking for the Needle in the Haystack?." *International Journal of Infectious Diseases* 89 (December 1, 2019): 146–53. https://doi.org/10.1016/j.ijid.2019.10.011.

Wilson, James M., V. "Signal Recognition during the Emergence of Pandemic Influenza Type A/H1N1: A Commercial Disease Intelligence Unit's Perspective." *Intelligence and National Security* 32, no. 2 (February 23, 2017): 222–30. https://doi.org/10.1080/02684527.2016.1253924.

Wilson, James M., Christopher K. Lake, Michael Matthews, Malinda Southard, Ryan M. Leone, and Maureen McCarthy. "Health Security Warning Intelligence During First Contact With COVID: An Operations Perspective." *Intelligence and National Security*, March 31, 2022, 1–24. https://doi.org/10.1080/02684527.2021.2020034.

Wilson, James M., Garrett M. Scalaro, and Jodie A. Powell. "Influenza Pandemic Warning Signals: Philadelphia in 1918 and 1977–1978." *Intelligence and National Security* 35, no. 4 (June 6, 2020): 502–18. https://doi.org/10.1080/02684527.2020.1750141.

Wirtz, James J. "COVID-19: Observations for Contemporary Strategists." *Defence Studies* 21, no. 2 (2021): 127–40. https://doi.org/10.1080/14702436.2021.1896361.

———. "Responding to Surprise." *Annual Review of Political Science* 9, no. 1 (May 15, 2006): 45–65. https://doi.org/10.1146/annurev.polisci.9.062404.170600.

World Economic Forum. "The Global Risks Report 2021: 16th Edition," 2021. https://www.weforum.org/reports/the-global-risks-report-2021.

Worobey, Michael, Jonathan Pekar, Brendan B. Larsen, Martha I. Nelson, Verity Hill, Jeffrey B. Joy, Andrew Rambaut, Marc A. Suchard, Joel O. Wertheim, and Philippe Lemey. "The Emergence of SARS-CoV-2 in Europe and North America." *Science* 370, no. 6516 (October 30, 2020): 564–70. https://doi.org/10.1126/science.abc8169.

Worwor, George, Anthony David Harries, Onofre Edwin Merilles Jr., Kerri Viney, Jean Jacques Rory, George Taleo, and Philippe Guyant. "Syndromic Surveillance in Vanuatu Since Cyclone Pam: A Descriptive Study." *Western Pacific Surveillance and Response Journal* 7, no. 4 (2016): 6–11. https://doi.org/10.5365/WPSAR.2016.7.3.009.

Yang, Weizhong, Zhongjie Li, Yajia Lan, Jinfeng Wang, Jiaqi Ma, Lianmei Jin, Qiao Sun, et al. "A Nationwide Web-Based Automated System for Outbreak Early Detection and Rapid Response in China." *Western Pacific Surveillance and Response Journal* 2, no. 1 (March 8, 2011): 10–15. https://doi.org/10.5365/WPSAR.2010.1.1.009.

Youde, Jeremy. *Globalization and Health.* Lanham, MD: Rowman & Littlefield, 2020.

Zegart, Amy B. *Spying Blind: The CIA, the FBI, and the Origins of 9/11.* Princeton, NJ: Princeton University Press, 2007.

Zhang, Ying, Hugo Lopez-Gatell, Celia M. Alpuche-Aranda, and Michael A. Stoto. "Did Advances in Global Surveillance and Notification Systems Make a Difference in the 2009 H1N1 Pandemic?—A Retrospective Analysis." *PLOS ONE* 8, no. 4 (April 3, 2013): e59893. https://doi.org/10.1371/journal.pone.0059893.

Zwald, Marissa L., Wen Lin, Gail L. Sondermeyer Cooksey, Charles Weiss, Angela Suarez, Marc Fischer, Brandon J. Bonin, et al. "Rapid Sentinel Surveillance for COVID-19—Santa Clara County, California, March 2020." *Morbidity and Mortality Weekly Report* 69, no. 14 (April 10, 2020): 419–21. https://doi.org/10.15585/mmwr .mm6914e3.

# INDEX

Note: Information in figures is indicated by page numbers in *italics*.

# ABOUT THE AUTHOR

ERIK J. DAHL is an associate professor of national security affairs at the Naval Postgraduate School in Monterey, California, where he is also on the faculty of the Center for Homeland Defense and Security. He is the author of *Intelligence and Surprise Attack: Failure and Success from Pearl Harbor to 9/11 and Beyond* (Georgetown University Press, 2013); his research and teaching focus on intelligence, terrorism, and international and homeland security. Dahl retired from the US Navy in 2002 after serving twenty-one years as an intelligence officer and received his PhD from the Fletcher School of Tufts University. He is a former chair of the Intelligence Studies Section of the International Studies Association.